Information Circular 9476

Analysis of Mine Fires for All U.S. Metal/Nonmetal Mining Categories,1990–2001

By Maria I. De Rosa

U.S. DEPARTMENT OF HEALTH AND HUMAN SERVICES
Centers for Disease Control and Prevention
National Institute for Occupational Safety and Health
Pittsburgh Research Laboratory
Pittsburgh, PA

November 2004

ORDERING INFORMATION

Copies of National Institute for Occupational Safety and Health (NIOSH)
documents and information
about occupational safety and health are available from

NIOSH–Publications Dissemination
4676 Columbia Parkway
Cincinnati, OH 45226–1998

FAX:	513–533–8573
Telephone:	1–800–35–NIOSH
	(1–800–356–4674)
E-mail:	pubstaft@cdc.gov
Web site:	www.cdc.gov/niosh

DHHS (NIOSH) Publication No. 2005–105

CONTENTS

CONTENTS–Continued

ILLUSTRATIONS

TABLES

TABLES–Continued

TABLES–Continued

UNIT OF MEASURE ABBREVIATIONS USED IN THIS REPORT

hr	hour(s)		st	short tons
min	minute(s)			

ANALYSIS OF MINE FIRES FOR ALL U.S. METAL/NONMETAL MINING CATEGORIES, 1990–2001

By Maria I. De Rosa[1]

ABSTRACT

This report analyzes mine fires for all U.S. underground and surface metal/nonmetal mining categories during 1990–2001 by state and six successive 2-year time periods. Injury risk rates are derived, and ignition source, methods of detection and suppression, and other variables are examined. Fires involving contractors are also included in the analysis. The data were derived from Mine Safety and Health Administration (MSHA) mine fire accident publications and verbal communications with mine personnel. The analysis will provide the National Institute for Occupational Safety and Health, MSHA, and the mining industry with a better understanding of the causes and hazards associated with mine fires and an increased awareness aimed at preventing and reducing fire hazards. It will also form a basis for future fire research programs.

[1]Industrial hygienist, Pittsburgh Research Laboratory, National Institute for Occupational Safety and Health, Pittsburgh, PA.

INTRODUCTION

Mine fires pose a constant danger to the safety of miners and to their livelihood. Underground mine fires pose an added hazard because of the confined environment with remote exits. Enactment of safety regulations [30 CFR[2] 56, 57] for underground and surface metal/nonmetal operations has greatly improved the safety of miners. However, mine fires and fire injuries remain serious hazards for all underground and surface mines.

This report analyzes mine fires and fire injuries for all U.S. metal/nonmetal mining categories, including sand and gravel and stone operations, during 1990–2001. Fires involving contractors are also included in the analysis. A similar analysis of fire incidents in metal/nonmetal mines during 1950–1984 was done by the former U.S. Bureau of Mines (USBM) [Butani and Pomroy 1987]. Detailed analyses of mobile equipment fires for all underground and surface coal and metal/nonmetal mining categories during 1990–1999 have recently been reported by NIOSH [De Rosa 2004].

Injury risk rate (Irr) values for the 12-year time period (1990–2001) and for six successive 2-year time periods within the 12-year period are derived. Irr values for individual states for the 12-year period are also derived. Other variables by state and time period include employees' working hours and lost workdays. The number of fire fatalities is reported by time period. Variables such as ignition source, method of detection and suppression, equipment involved, location, and burning material are reported by six 2-year time periods only. Further-more, the number of fire injuries per number of fires causing injuries and total fires has been analyzed by year, ignition source, equipment involved, and location. For comparison purposes, the major fire and fire injury findings for all metal/nonmetal mining categories have been reported.

The data in this report were derived from "Injury Experience" publications [MSHA 1991a,b,c,d; 1992a,b,c,d; 1993a,b,c,d; 1994a,b,c,d; 1995a,b,c,d; 1996a,b,c,d; 1997a,b,c,d; 1998a,b,c,d; 1999a,b,c,d; 2000a,b,c,d; 2001a,b,c,d; 2002a,b,c,d], "Fire Accident Reports" [MSHA 1993e; 1994e; 1995e; 1996e; 1997e,f; 2000e], MSHA "Fire Accident Abstracts" internal publications, and verbal communications with mine personnel. Mining companies are required by 30 CFR 50 to report to MSHA all fires that result in injuries and fires that are not extinguished within 30 min of discovery. A small number of fires lasting <30 min without injuries reported in the "Fire Accident Abstracts" have been included in this report. Also included in this report are fires caused by explosions and explosives.

The analysis in this report will provide the National Institute for Occupational Safety and Health (NIOSH), the Mine Safety and Health Administration (MSHA), and the mining industry with a better understanding of the causes and hazards of mine fires and fire injuries and an increased awareness aimed at preventing and reducing fire hazards. It will also form a basis for developing future fire research programs.

METHODOLOGIES

For all metal/nonmetal mining categories, data on mine fires during 1990–2001 have been reported as actual numbers and calculated values.

1. For each mining category, actual numbers include the total number of fires, fire injuries, employees' working hours, and lost workdays for a 12-year period (1990–2001) and for six successive 2-year periods within the 12-year period. These numbers have also been reported by state for the 12-year time period. The actual number of fire fatalities has been reported by time period. Furthermore, actual numbers of fires for the six 2-year periods have been reported by ignition source, method of detection and suppression, equipment involved, location, and burning material. Actual numbers of fire injuries per number of fires causing injuries and total fires have been reported by year, ignition source, equipment involved, and location.

2. For each mining category, the calculated values include the injury risk rates during the 12-year period and the six 2-year periods. The injury risk rate (Irr) values were calculated according to the MSHA formula (incidence rate (IR) = number of fire injuries × 200,000 working hours divided by the total employees' working hours) [MSHA 1991a,b,c,d; 1992a,b,c,d; 1993a,b,c,d; 1994a,b,c,d; 1995a,b,c,d; 1996a,b,c,d; 1997a,b,c,d; 1998a,b,c,d; 1999a,b,c,d; 2000a,b,c,d; 2001a,b,c,d; 2002a,b,c,d]. Also, injury risk rate values for individual states (12-year period) were calculated according to this same formula.

For comparison purposes, only the injury risk rate values for 12-year and 2-year time periods and the injury risk rate values for individual states (12-year time period) with the highest number of fire injuries have been considered. The fatality risk rate values have not been calculated because of the small number of fatalities that occurred during the 12-year period.

3. Calculations of Irr values are as follows:

a. Injury risk rate (Irr) value: Number of fire injuries × 200,000 working hours divided by total employees' working hours. The Irr value is the average risk rate value for the number of fire injuries per 200,000 working hours for a given time period.

b. Total employees' working hour (Ewhr) value during 1990–2001: Sum of 12 yearly Ewhr values for all of the

---

[2]*Code of Federal Regulations.* See CFR in references.

states involved in fires. This value also includes the Ewhr value reported for all other states not involved in fires. The Ewhr value for each state (12-year time period) is the sum of 12 yearly Ewhr values for that state.

c. Total employees' working hours (Ewhr) value for six 2-year time periods: Sum of two yearly Ewhr values for all of the states involved and not involved in fires within the 2-year period.

d. The lost workday (LWD) values were reported by state and time period.

e. A lost workday value of 6,000, assigned by MSHA to each fatality or permanent total disability, was reported.

FIRE DATA ANALYSIS FOR ALL METAL/NONMETAL MINING CATEGORIES

UNDERGROUND METAL/NONMETAL AND STONE MINE FIRES

Table 1 and figure 1 show the number of fires and fire injuries that occurred in underground metal/nonmetal and stone mines by state during 1990–2001. Table 1 also shows the injury risk rates, employees' working hours, and lost workdays. Overall, 65 fires occurred in 20 states; these include 2 fires and no injuries for contractors. Six of the fires caused nine injuries. The yearly average was 5.4 fires and 0.75 injury. Forty-one fires with 2 injuries occurred in metal mines, 14 fires with 7 injuries occurred in nonmetal mines, and 10 fires with no injuries occurred in stone mines. The underground mine fires required 25 mine rescue team interventions and 30 mine/section evacuations. The Ewhr value was 260×10^6 hr (Irr = 0.007), and the LWD value was 83.

Idaho had the most fires (eight fires and no injuries), followed by Louisiana (seven fires and two injuries), Michigan (six fires and six injuries), and Missouri (six fires and no injuries). Of these states, Michigan had the highest injury risk rate value (Irr = 0.146).

Table 2, partly illustrated in figure 2, shows the number of fires, fire injuries, risk rates, employees' working hours, and lost workdays by time period. The number of fires during the six time periods show an increase during the fourth period followed by a sharp decrease during the fifth period and a sharp increase in the last period. The number of fire injuries show an increase followed by a decrease during most of the periods, accompanied by a decline in employees' working hours during most of the periods; an increase is seen during the third and fourth periods. The Irr values follow patterns similar to those shown by the injury values.

Tables 3–8 show the number of fires by ignition source, method of detection and suppression, equipment involved, location, and burning material by time period. Figure 3 shows the major variables related to fires for 1990–2001. Table 9 shows the number of fire injuries per number of fires causing injuries and total fires by year, ignition source, equipment involved, and location.

Ignition Source

Table 3 shows the number of fires by ignition source for each time period. The sources that caused most of the underground metal/nonmetal and stone mine fires were hydraulic fluid/fuel sprayed onto equipment hot surfaces (16 fires or 25%), flame cutting/welding spark/slag/flame (13 fires or 20%), and electrical short/arcing (12 fires or 19%).

Thirteen of the 16 mobile equipment hydraulic fluid/fuel fires became large fires because of the continuous flow of fluids from the pumps due to engine shutoff failure, lack of an emergency line drainage system, or lack of effective and rapid local firefighting response capabilities. In at least two instances during these fires, the cab was suddenly engulfed in flames, probably due to the ignition of flammable vapors and mists that penetrated the cab. Of note is that the hydraulic fluid fires subsequently involved the fuel system. Other ignition sources included engine/motor mechanical malfunctions, spontaneous combustion (involving timber)/hot material, conveyor belt/equipment friction, heat source (mostly involving heaters), overheated oil, and explosion/ignition of explosives. Fires caused by the spontaneous combustion/hot material and electrical short/arcing ignition sources were usually detected long after they had started due to lack of combustion gas/smoke detection systems.

During the first period, the largest number of fires were caused by hydraulic fluid/fuel sprayed onto equipment hot surfaces, flame cutting/welding spark/slag/flame, and electrical short/arcing sources. During the second period, the largest number of fires were caused by flame cutting/welding spark/slag/flame and electrical short/arcing sources. During the third period, the largest number of fires were caused by conveyor belt/equipment friction. During the fourth period, the largest number of fires were caused by hydraulic fluid/fuel sprayed onto equipment hot surfaces. During the fifth period, the largest number of fires were caused by hydraulic fluid/fuel sprayed onto equipment hot surfaces and flame cutting/welding spark/slag/flame. During the sixth period, the largest number of fires were caused by hydraulic fluid/fuel.

Method of Detection

Table 4 shows the number of fires by method of detection for each time period. The most frequent methods were miners who saw smoke long after the fire had started, operators who saw the fires when they started as flames/flash fires, and miners who saw smoke shortly after the fires had started. Other methods of detection were welders who saw sparks, miners who heard an explosion or smelled smoke, and operators who experienced an equipment power loss. One fire was detected by carbon monoxide gas sampling, and two fires were undetected.

During the first period, the largest number of fires were detected by operators as flames/flash fires. During the second period, the largest number of fires were detected by welders as sparks. During the third, fifth, and sixth periods, the largest number of fires were detected by miners as smoke long after the fires had started. During the fourth period, the largest number of fires were detected visually as flames and sparks.

Table 1.—Number of fires, fire injuries, and risk rates for underground metal/nonmetal
and stone mines by state, employees' working hours, and lost workdays, 1990–2001

State[1]	No. fires[1]	No. fire injuries[1]	LWD[2]	Ewhr,[2] 10^6 hr	Irr[3]
Alaska	1	—	—	2	—
Arizona	3	—	—	28.3	—
Colorado	3	—	—	9.6	—
Idaho	8	—	—	9.7	—
Illinois	2	—	—	0.5	—
Indiana	2	—	—	2.1	—
Kansas	1	—	—	1	—
Kentucky	2	—	—	11.3	—
Louisiana	7	2	24	7.4	0.054
Michigan	6	6	52	8.2	0.146
Missouri	6	—	—	16.8	—
Montana	2	—	—	10.5	—
Nevada	3	—	—	14	—
New Mexico	4	—	—	22.8	—
New York	5	—	—	9.4	—
Ohio	2	—	—	5.7	—
South Dakota	3	—	—	12.1	—
Tennessee	1	—	—	14	—
Washington	1	—	—	3	—
Wyoming	3	1	7	24.5	0.008
All other states	—	—	—	47	—
Total	65	9	83	260	[3]0.007

[1]Derived from MSHA "Fire Accident Abstract" internal publications.
[2]Derived from MSHA "Injury Experience in Mining" publications.
[3]Calculated according to MSHA formula reported in the "Methodologies" section.

Table 2.—Number of fires, fire injuries, and risk rates for underground metal/nonmetal and stone mines
by time period, employees' working hours, and lost workdays, 1990–2001

	Time period						1990-2001
	90-91	92-93	94-95	96-97	98-99	00-01	
Number of fires[1]	10	10	10	15	6	14	65
Number of fire injuries[1]	1	3	—	5	—	—	9
LWD[2]	2	31	—	50	—	—	83
Ewhr,[2] 10^6 hr	49	42	43	45	41	40	260
Irr[3]	0.004	0.014	—	0.022	—	—	[3]0.007

[1]Derived from MSHA "Fire Accident Abstract" internal publications.
[2]Derived from MSHA "Injury Experience in Mining" publications.
[3]Calculated according to MSHA formula reported in the "Methodologies" section.

Table 3.—Number of fires for underground metal/nonmetal and stone mines by ignition source and time period,
1990–2001

Ignition source	Time period						1990-2001
	90-91 No. fires	92-93 No. fires	94-95 No. fires	96-97 No. fires	98-99 No. fires	00-01 No. fires	No. fires
Hydraulic fluid/fuel on equipment hot surfaces	2	2	2	4	2	4	16
Flame cutting/welding spark/slag/flame	2	3	2	3	2	1	13
Electrical short/arcing	2	3	1	1	1	4	12
Engine/motor malfunction	—	1	—	3	—	1	5
Conveyor belt/equipment friction	—	—	3	2	—	—	5
Spontaneous combustion (involving timber)/ hot material	1	1	—	—	—	3	5
Heat source	1	—	1	—	1	1	4
Explosion/ignition-explosives	1	—	1	—	—	—	2
Overheated oil	—	—	—	2	—	—	2
Unknown	1	—	—	—	—	—	1
Total	10	10	10	15	6	14	65

Table 4.—Number of fires for underground metal/nonmetal and stone mines by method of detection and time period, 1990–2001

Method of detection	Time period						
	90-91 No. fires	92-93 No. fires	94-95 No. fires	96-97 No. fires	98-99 No. fires	00-01 No. fires	1990-2001 No. fires
Visual:							
Late smoke detection	1	2	4	2	3	6	18
Flames/flash fires	3	2	3	3	2	4	17
Sparks	2	3	1	3	1	—	10
Heard explosion	1	—	1	—	—	—	3
Smelled smoke	—	1	—	—	—	1	2
Power loss	—	1	—	—	—	—	1
CO gas sampling	—	1	—	—	—	—	1
Undetected	2	—	—	—	—	—	2
Total	10	10	10	15	6	14	65

Table 5.—Number of fires for underground metal/nonmetal and stone mines by suppression method and time period, 1990–2001

Suppression method	Time period						
	90-91 No. fires	92-93 No. fires	94-95 No. fires	96-97 No. fires	98-99 No. fires	00-01 No. fires	1990-2001 No. fires
FE-DCP-foam-water	2	4	2	3	3	9	23
Water	3	3	2	4	3	3	18
Portable fire extinguisher	3	2	1	6	—	2	14
FSS-DCP-foam-water	—	1	1	—	—	—	2
FSS-HD[1]	—	—	1	1	—	—	2
Manual with FE[2]	—	—	1	—	—	—	1
Destroyed/HD[3]	2	—	2	1	—	—	5
Total	10	10	10	15	6	14	65

DCP   Dry chemical powder.
FE   Portable fire extinguisher.
FSS   Machine fire suppression system.
HD   Heavily damaged.
[1]Heavy damage to equipment due to FSS activation failure or late activation.
[2]Method used by welders to extinguish clothing and oxyfuel/grease fires.
[3]Usually due to failure of other firefighting methods, late fire detection, undetected fires, or fire size.

Table 6.—Number of fires for underground metal/nonmetal and stone mines by equipment involved and time period, 1990–2001

Equipment	Time period						
	90-91 No. fires	92-93 No. fires	94-95 No. fires	96-97 No. fires	98-99 No. fires	00-01 No. fires	1990-2001 No. fires
Mobile equipment[1]	3	5	4	9	3	7	31
Oxyfuel torch[2]	2	3	1	2	2	—	10
Beltline	—	—	3	1	—	1	5
Electrical system/battery/charger	1	1	—	—	—	3	5
Heater/cutting saw	1	—	—	1	1	1	4
Explosive box	1	—	1	—	—	—	2
Air compressor	—	—	—	2	—	—	2
Other[3]	2	1	1	—	—	2	6
Total	10	10	10	15	6	14	65

[1]Includes golf and ore carts, locomotives, loaders, scoops, tractors, shuttle cars, power scalers, trolleys, trucks, and drills.
[2]At times, electrical arc welding equipment was used.
[3]Did not involve equipment.

Table 7.—Number of fires for underground metal/nonmetal and stone mines by location and time period, 1990–2001

Location	Time period						
	90-91 No. fires	92-93 No. fires	94-95 No. fires	96-97 No. fires	98-99 No. fires	00-01 No. fires	1990-2001 No. fires
Mobile equipment working areas[1]	3	4	2	6	1	4	20
Flame cutting/welding areas[2]	2	3	2	3	2	1	13
Mine face/section/crosscut/drift areas	2	2	—	2	—	1	7
Battery/motor barn/pipeline areas	1	—	1	1	1	2	6
Belt entry	—	—	3	1	—	1	5
Shop/refuse/maintenance areas	1	—	—	—	1	2	4
Chute/crusher/air compressor areas	—	—	1	1	—	1	3
Decline slopes	—	1	—	—	1	1	3
Gobline/abandoned areas	1	—	—	—	—	1	2
Panel/tunnel areas	—	—	1	1	—	—	2
Total	10	10	10	15	6	14	65

[1]Includes haulage, loading, mucking, transportation, and drilling areas.
[2]Includes shops, mainways, boreholes, shafts, stations, slusher buckets and chute areas, and mobile equipment maintenance areas.

Table 8.—Number of fires for underground metal/nonmetal and stone mines by burning material and time period, 1990–2001

Burning material	Time period						
	90-91 No. fires	92-93 No. fires	94-95 No. fires	96-97 No. fires	98-99 No. fires	00-01 No. fires	1990-2001 No. fires
Hydraulic fluid/fuel	2	2	2	4	2	4	16
Electrical cord/cables/wires/batteries	3	3	1	1	1	4	13
Oxyfuel/clothing/grease/other[1]	2	3	2	3	2	1	13
Belt material	—	—	3	2	—	1	6
Refueling fuel/flammable liquid/oil/ grease/refuse	2	—	1	2	1	—	6
Timber/pipeline/chute liner	—	1	—	—	—	3	4
Equipment mechanical components	—	1	—	3	—	—	4
Detonated explosives	1	—	1	—	—	—	2
Shop/content	—	—	—	—	—	1	1
Total	10	10	10	15	6	14	65

[1]Includes rubber tires and hoses, refuse, chute liner, hydraulic fluid, shop, wood, and shaft material.

Table 9.—Number of fire injuries per number of fires causing injuries and total fires for underground metal/nonmetal and stone mines by year, ignition source, equipment involved, and location, 1990–2001

Year	No. total fires	No. fires causing injuries	No. fire injuries	Ignition source	Equipment	Location
1990	3	1	1	Hydraulic fluid/fuel on equipment hot surfaces	Ore cart	Transportation area.
1991	7	—	—	—	—	—
1992	6	2	1	Flame cutting/welding spark/slag/flame	Oxyfuel torch	Flame cutting/welding areas.
			1	Overheated oil	Scoop	Mining area.
1993	4	1	1	Flame cutting/welding spark/slag/flame	Oxyfuel torch	Flame cutting/welding areas.
1994	8	—	—	—	—	—
1995	2	—	—	—	—	—
1996	6	1	1	Overheated oil	Air compressor	Drilling area.
1997	9	1	4	Hydraulic fluid/fuel on equipment hot surfaces	Scoop	Mining area.
1998	3	—	—	—	—	—
1999	3	—	—	—	—	—
2000	8	—	—	—	—	—
2001	6	—	—	—	—	—
Total	65	6	9			

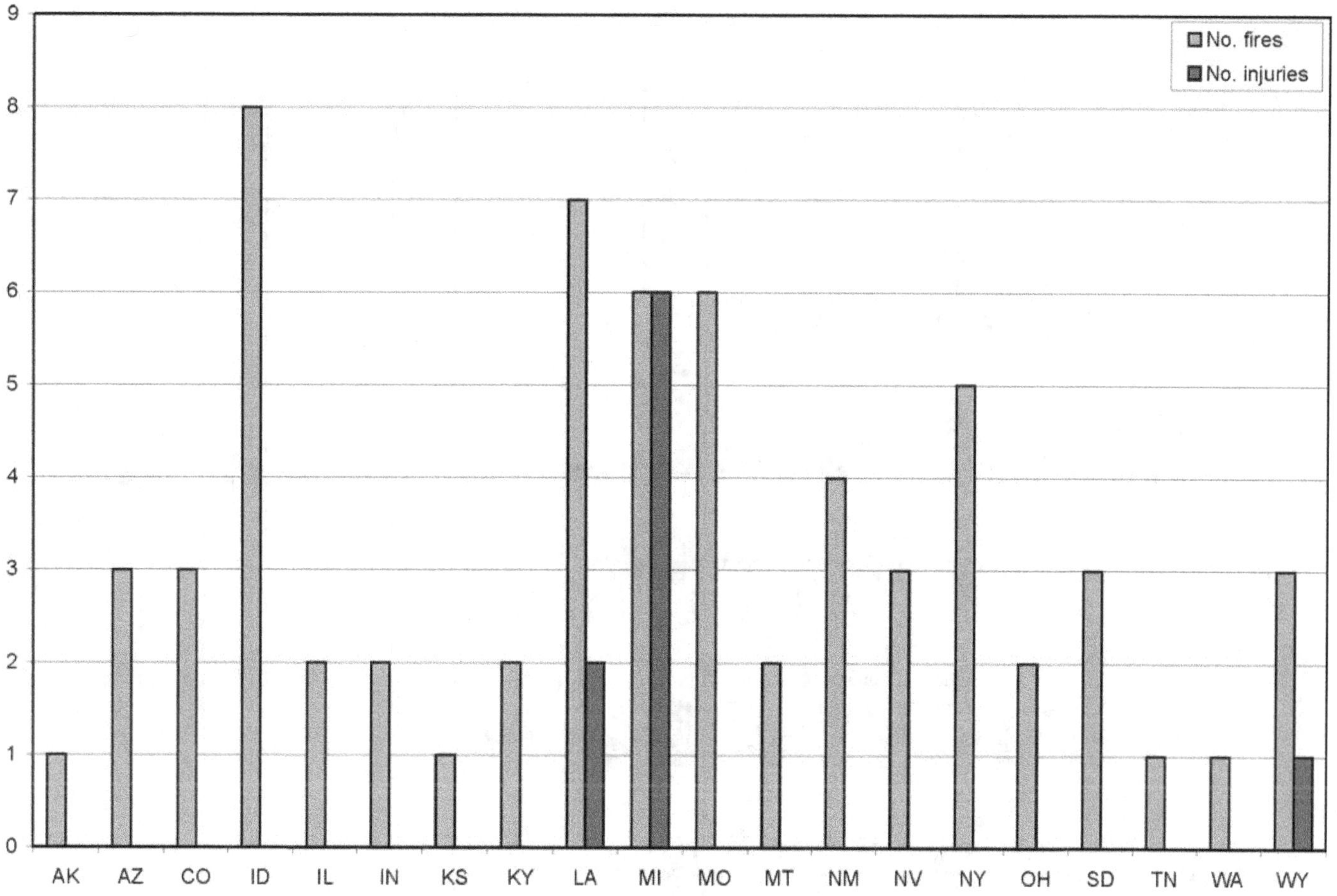

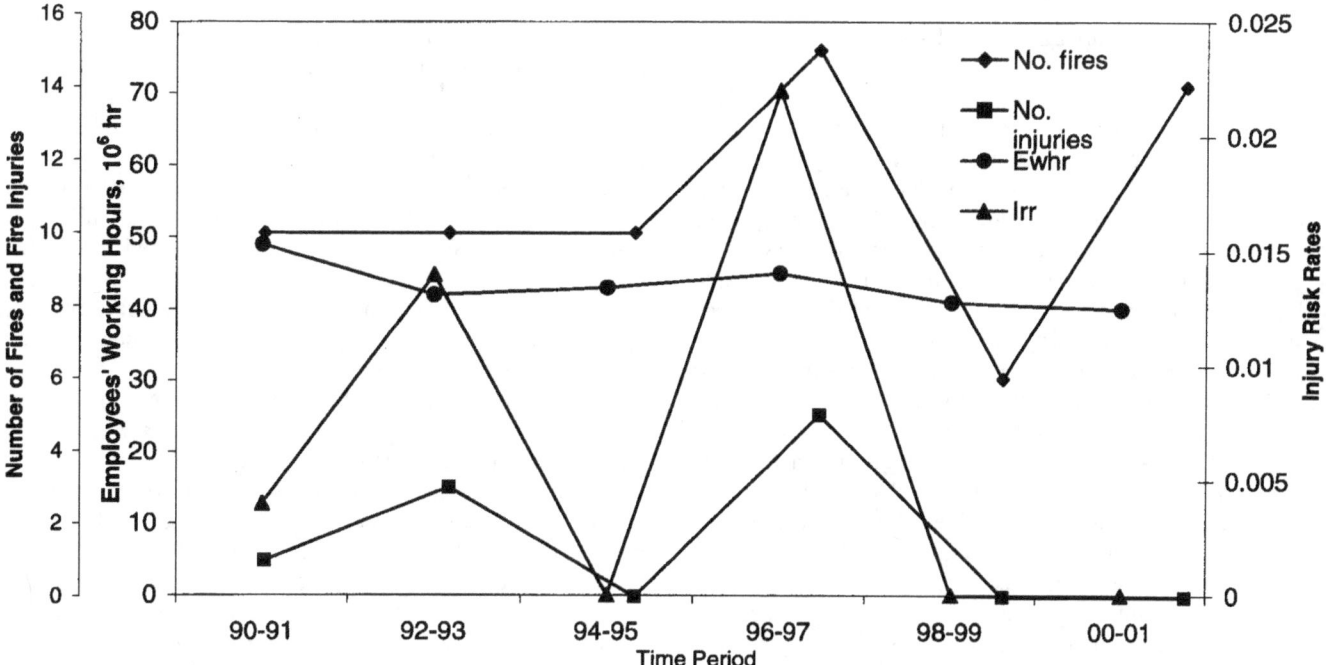

Figure 1.—Number of fires and fire injuries for underground metal/nonmetal and stone mines by state, 1990–2001.

Figure 2.—Number of fires, fire injuries, risk rates, and employees' working hours for underground metal/nonmetal and stone mines by time period, 1990–2001.

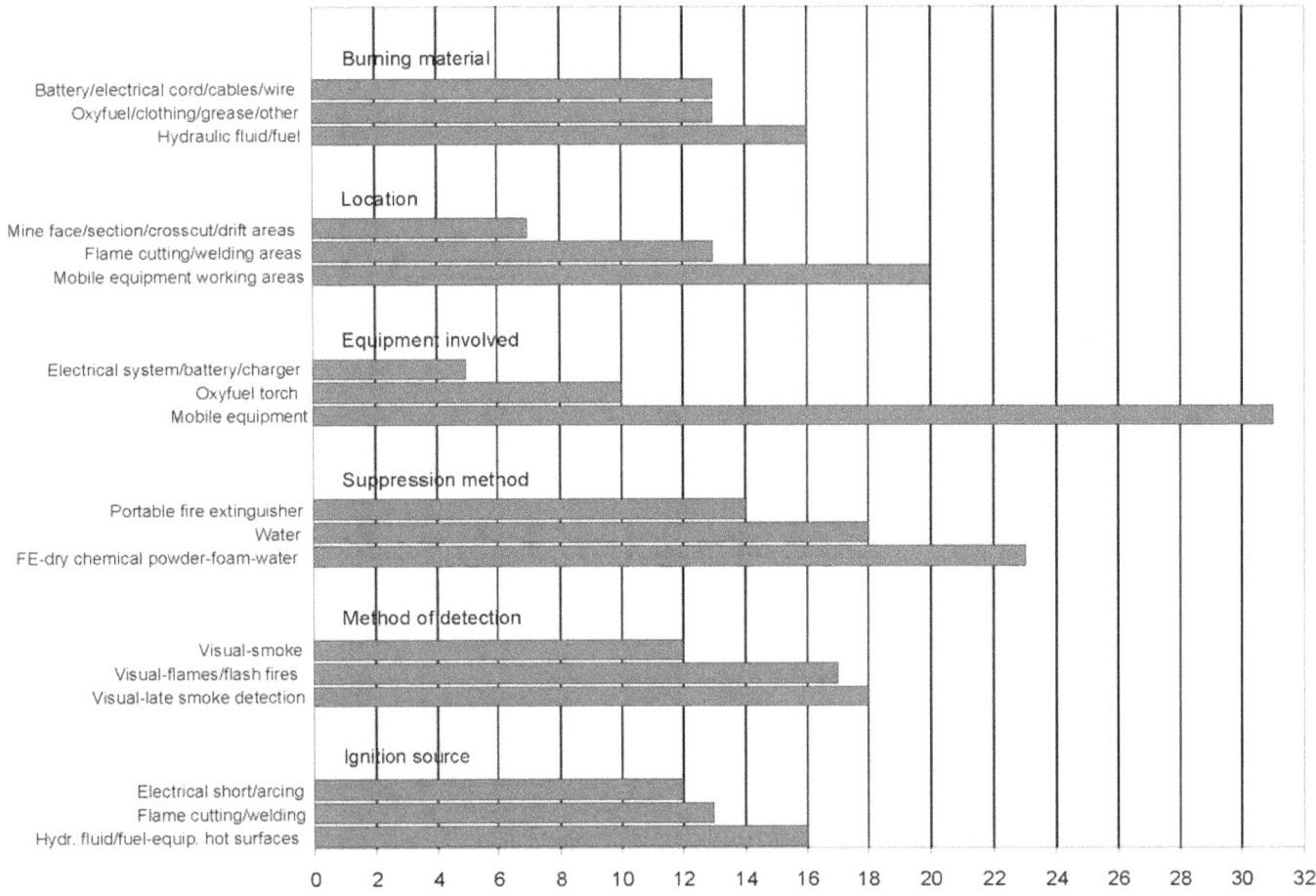

Figure 3.—Major variables for underground metal/nonmetal and stone mine fires, 1990–2001. (FE = portable fire extinguisher)

Suppression Method

Table 5 shows the number of fires by suppression method for each time period. Usually more than one agent was used to fight a fire. The most common methods were portable fire extinguishers with dry chemical powder, foam, and water, followed by water or portable fire extinguishers alone. Other suppression methods included machine fire suppression systems with dry chemical powder, foam, and water and manual techniques with or without portable fire extinguishers (welders' method to extinguish clothing and oxyfuel/grease fires). Four of the 16 pieces of mobile equipment involved in hydraulic fluid/fuel fires had machine fire suppression systems. Dual activations (two activations) of machine fire suppression and engine shutoff systems succeeded in temporarily abating the fires; however, the flames reignited, fueled by the flow of pressurized fluids entrapped in the lines. On one occasion the fire suppression system failed to activate, and in another instance the system was activated late.

Portable fire extinguishers, used upon discovery of the fires, were successful in extinguishing small fires involving oxyfuel/ grease, oil, refueling fuel, and electrical wires, cables and batteries. Mine rescue teams (required 25 times), upon mine/ section evacuation (performed 30 times), fought the fires (including 12 mobile equipment fires) with dry chemical powder and water; in one instance, foam was also used. However, seven fires destroyed or heavily damaged equipment (including four pieces of mobile equipment) because of failure of firefighting methods, late fire detection, undetected fires, or fire size. Other factors that determined the success of fire suppression efforts were the time lapse between detection and application of extinguishing agents and effective and rapid local firefighting response capabilities.

During the first period, the largest number of fires were suppressed with portable fire extinguishers or water alone. During the second and sixth periods, the largest number of fires were suppressed with portable fire extinguishers together with dry chemical powder, foam, and water. During the third and fifth periods, the largest number of fires were suppressed with water alone and portable fire extinguishers with dry chemical powder, foam, and water. During the fourth period, the largest number of fires were suppressed with portable fire extinguishers alone.

Equipment Involved

Table 6 shows the number of fires by equipment involved for each time period. The equipment most often involved was mobile equipment (golf and ore carts, locomotives, shuttle cars, loaders, power scalers, scoops, tractors, trolleys, trucks, and drills), followed by oxyfuel torches (at times electrical arc welding equipment was used). Other equipment included belt-lines, electrical systems, batteries, chargers, heaters, cutting saws, explosive boxes, and air compressors. Six fires did not involve equipment. During all of the periods, the largest number of fires involved mobile equipment.

Location

Table 7 shows the number of fires by location for each time period. The most common locations were mobile equipment working areas (haulage, loading, mucking, transportation and drilling areas, decline slopes), followed by flame cutting/welding areas (at shops, mainways, boreholes, shafts, stations, slusher bucket and chute areas, and maintenance areas), and mine face, section, crosscut, and drift areas. Other fire locations were battery and pipeline areas, motor barns, belt entries, shops, refuse and maintenance areas, decline slopes, chute and crusher areas, panel and tunnel areas, and goblines and abandoned areas.

During the first, second, fourth, and sixth periods, the largest number of fires occurred at mobile equipment working areas. During the third period, the largest number of fires occurred at belt entries. During the fifth period, the largest number of fires occurred at flame cutting/welding areas.

Burning Materials

Table 8 shows the number of fires by burning material for each time period. The materials most often involved were hydraulic fluid/fuel, electrical cord, cables, wires, batteries, oxyfuel/clothing/grease, and materials such as rubber tires and hoses, hydraulic fluid, shop, refuse, wood, chute liner, and shaft material. Other burning materials included belt material, refueling fuel, flammable liquids, oil, grease, refuse, timber, pipelines, chute liners, equipment mechanical components, detonated explosives, and shops and their content.

During the first period, the largest number of fires involved electrical cord, cables, wires, and batteries. During the second period, the largest number of fires involved oxyfuel, clothing/grease, and other materials and electrical cord, cables, wires, and batteries. During the third period, the largest number of fires involved belt materials. During the fourth period, the largest number of fires involved hydraulic fluid/fuel. During the fifth period, the largest number of fires involved hydraulic fluid/fuel and oxyfuel. During the sixth period, the largest number of fires involved hydraulic fluid/fuel and electrical materials.

Fire Injuries

Table 9 shows the number of fire injuries per number of fires causing injuries and total fires by year, ignition source, equipment involved, and location during 1990–2001. Overall, there were nine injuries caused by six fires. The greatest number of fire injuries occurred in 1997 (four injuries caused by one fire). The ignition sources that caused the fire injuries were hydraulic fluid/fuel sprayed onto equipment hot surfaces, flame cutting/welding spark/slag/flame, and overheated oil. The equipment involved in fire injuries included mobile equipment, oxyfuel torches, and air compressors. The locations where the fire injuries occurred were mobile equipment working areas, flame cutting/welding areas, and mining areas.

SURFACE OF UNDERGROUND METAL/NONMETAL AND STONE MINE FIRES

Table 10 and figure 4 show the number of fires and fire injuries occurring at the surface of underground metal/nonmetal and stone mines by state during 1990–2001. Table 10 also shows the injury risk rates, employees' working hours, and lost workdays.

A total of 12 fires occurred in 11 states; 5 of the fires caused 5 injuries. The yearly average was one fire and 0.42 injury. Five fires with two injuries occurred at metal mines, five fires with two injuries occurred at nonmetal mines, and two fires with one injury occurred at stone mines. None of the fires involved contractors. The Ewhr value was 58×10^6 hr (Irr = 0.017), and the LWD value was 75.

Nevada had the most fires (two fires and no injuries). Ohio, New Mexico, Missouri, South Dakota, and Idaho each had one fire with one injury. Of these states, Missouri had the highest injury risk rate value (Irr = 0.25).

Table 11, partly illustrated in figure 5, shows the number of fires, fire injuries, risk rates, employees' working hours, and lost workdays by time period. The number of fires decreased during most of the six time periods. The number of fire injuries and employees' working hours decreased during all of the periods. The Irr values follow patterns similar to those shown by the injury values.

Tables 12–17 show the number of fires by ignition source, method of detection and suppression, equipment involved, location, and burning material by time period. Figure 6 shows the major variables related to fires for 1990–2001. Table 18 shows the number of fire injuries per number of fires causing injuries and total fires by year, ignition source, equipment involved, and location.

Ignition Source

Table 12 shows the number of fires and fire injuries by ignition source for each time period. The leading source was flame cutting/welding spark/slag/flame (seven fires or 58%), followed by electrical short/arcing and heat source (one fire for each ignition). The ignition sources for three fires were unknown.

During the first through third periods, the fires were caused by the flame cutting/welding spark/slag/flame source. During the fifth period, the fire was caused by a heat source. During the sixth period, the fires were caused by flame cutting/welding spark/slag/flame and electrical short/arcing sources. No fires occurred during the fourth period.

Method of Detection

Table 13 shows the number of fires by method of detection for each time period. The most frequent method was welders who saw sparks. This was followed by miners who saw smoke long after the fires had started and miners who saw smoke shortly after the fires had started. Three fires were undetected.

During the first period, the largest number of fires were detected by welders as sparks. During subsequent periods, the fires were detected by welders as sparks (second period), by miners as smoke shortly or long after the fires had started and by welders as sparks (third period), by miners as smoke (fifth period), and by welders and miners as sparks and as smoke (sixth period).

Table 10.—Number of fires, fire injuries, and risk rates for surface of underground metal/nonmetal and stone mines by state, employees' working hours, and lost workdays, 1990–2001

State[1]	No. fires[1]	No. fire injuries[1]	LWD[2]	Ewhr,[2] 10^6 hr	Irr[3]
California	1	—	—	0.7	—
Idaho	1	1	10	2.43	0.082
Kansas	1	—	—	0.26	—
Kentucky	1	—	—	3.1	—
Missouri	1	1	21	0.8	0.25
Montana	1	—	—	4	—
Nevada	2	—	—	3.1	—
New Mexico	1	1	16	2.6	0.077
Ohio	1	1	15	2.1	0.095
South Dakota	1	1	13	4	0.05
Utah	1	—	—	0.7	—
All other states	—	—	—	34.21	—
Total	12	5	75	58	[3]0.017

[1]Derived from MSHA "Fire Accident Abstract" internal publications.
[2]Derived from MSHA "Injury Experience in Mining" publications.
[3]Calculated according to MSHA formula reported in the "Methodologies" section.

Table 11.—Number of fires, fire injuries, and risk rates for surface of underground metal/nonmetal and stone mines by time period, employees' working hours, and lost workdays, 1990–2001

	Time period						1990-2001
	90-91	92-93	94-95	96-97	98-99	00-01	
Number of fires[1]	3	2	3	—	2	2	12
Number of fire injuries[1]	2	1	1	—	—	1	5
LWD[2]	16	—	56	—	—	3	75
Ewhr,[2] 10^6 hr	12	11	10	9	8	8	58
Irr[3]	0.033	0.018	0.02	—	—	0.025	[3]0.017

[1]Derived from MSHA "Fire Accident Abstract" internal publications.
[2]Derived from MSHA "Injury Experience in Mining" publications.
[3]Calculated according to MSHA formula reported in the "Methodologies" section.

Table 12.—Number of fires for surface of underground metal/nonmetal and stone mines by ignition source and time period, 1990–2001

Ignition source	Time period						1990-2001
	90-91 No. fires	92-93 No. fires	94-95 No. fires	96-97 No. fires	98-99 No. fires	00-01 No. fires	No. fires
Flame cutting/welding spark/slag/flame	2	1	3	—	—	1	7
Electrical short/arcing	—	—	—	—	—	1	1
Heat source	—	—	—	—	1	—	1
Unknown	1	1	—	—	1	—	3
Total	3	2	3	—	2	2	12

Table 13.—Number of fires for surface of underground metal/nonmetal and stone mines by method of detection and time period, 1990–2001

Method of detection	Time period						
	90-91 No. fires	92-93 No. fires	94-95 No. fires	96-97 No. fires	98-99 No. fires	00-01 No. fires	1990-2001 No. fires
Visual:							
Sparks	2	1	1	—	—	1	5
Smoke	—	—	1	—	—	1	2
Late smoke detection	—	—	1	—	1	—	2
Undetected	1	1	—	—	1	—	3
Total	3	2	3	—	2	2	12

Table 14.—Number of fires for surface of underground metal/nonmetal and stone mines by suppression method and time period, 1990–2001

Suppression method	Time period						
	90-91 No. fires	92-93 No. fires	94-95 No. fires	96-97 No. fires	98-99 No. fires	00-01 No. fires	1990-2001 No. fires
Water	—	—	2	—	1	1	4
Manual with or without FE[1]	2	—	1	—	—	—	3
FE	—	1	—	—	—	1	2
Destroyed/HD[2]	1	1	—	—	1	—	3
Total	3	2	3	—	2	2	12

FE   Portable fire extinguisher.
HD   Heavily damaged.
[1]Method used by welders to extinguish clothing and oxyfuel/grease fires.
[2]Usually due to failure of firefighting methods, undetected fires, or fire size.

Table 15.—Number of fires for surface of underground metal/nonmetal and stone mines by equipment involved and time period, 1990–2001

Equipment	Time period						
	90-91 No. fires	92-93 No. fires	94-95 No. fires	96-97 No. fires	98-99 No. fires	00-01 No. fires	1990-2001 No. fires
Oxyfuel torch[1]	2	1	3	—	—	1	7
Facilities[2]	1	1	—	—	1	1	3
Ventilation fan	—	—	—	—	—	1	1
Heater	—	—	—	—	1	—	1
Total	3	2	3	—	2	2	12

[1]At times, electrical arc welding equipment was used.
[2]Considered equipment in this report.

Table 16.—Number of fires for surface of underground metal/nonmetal and stone mines by location and time period, 1990–2001

Location	Time period						
	90-91 No. fires	92-93 No. fires	94-95 No. fires	96-97 No. fires	98-99 No. fires	00-01 No. fires	1990-2001 No. fires
Flame cutting/welding areas[1]	2	1	3	—	—	1	7
Facility/garage/trailer/storage areas	1	1	—	—	2	—	4
Fan housing	—	—	—	—	—	1	1
Total	3	2	3	—	2	2	12

[1]Includes shop, junction box, facilities, handrail, head frame, walkway, and maintenance areas.

Table 17.—Number of fires for surface of underground metal/nonmetal and stone mines by burning material and time period, 1990–2001

Burning material	Time period						
	90-91 No. fires	92-93 No. fires	94-95 No. fires	96-97 No. fires	98-99 No. fires	00-01 No. fires	1990-2001 No. fires
Oxyfuel/clothing/grease/other[1]	2	1	3	—	—	1	7
Facility/content	1	1	—	—	1	—	3
Wood	—	—	—	—	1	1	2
Total	3	2	3	—	2	2	12

[1]Includes electrical junction boxes, handrails, grease, flammable liquids, rubber tires, and equipment mechanical components.

Table 18.—Number of fire injuries per number of fires causing injuries and total fires for surface of underground metal/nonmetal and stone mines by year, ignition source, equipment involved, and location, 1990–2001

Year	No. total fires	No. fires causing injuries	No. fire injuries	Ignition source	Equipment	Location
1990	2	1	1	Flame cutting/welding spark/slag/flame	Oxyfuel torch ...	Flame cutting/welding areas.
1991	1	1	1	Flame cutting/welding spark/slag/flame	Oxyfuel torch ...	Flame cutting/welding areas.
1992	1	—	—	—	—	—
1993	1	1	1	Flame cutting/welding spark/slag/flame	Oxyfuel torch ...	Flame cutting/welding areas.
1994	2	1	1	Flame cutting/welding spark/slag/flame	Oxyfuel torch ...	Flame cutting/welding areas.
1995	1	—	—	—	—	—
1996	—	—	—	—	—	—
1997	—	—	—	—	—	—
1998	1	—	—	—	—	—
1999	1	—	—	—	—	—
2000	2	1	1	Flame cutting/welding spark/slag/flame	Oxyfuel torch ...	Flame cutting/welding areas.
2001	—	—	—	—	—	—
Total	12	5	5			

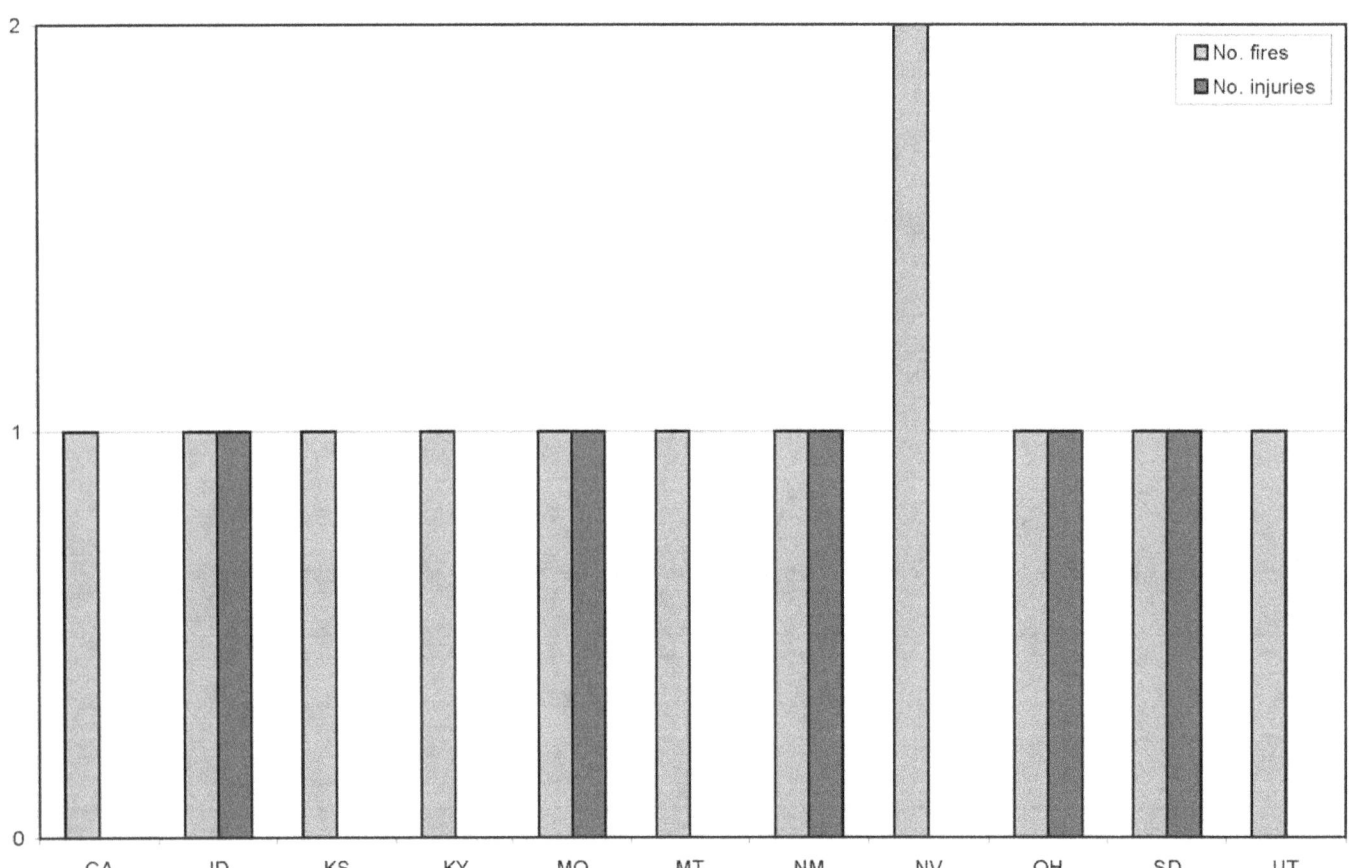

Figure 4.—Number of fires and fire injuries for surface of underground metal/nonmetal and stone mines by state, 1990–2001.

No. fires
No. injuries
Ewhr
Irr
Number of Fires and Fire Injuries
Employees' Working Hours, 10^6 hr
Injury Risk Rates
Time period
90-91
92-93
94-95
96-97
98-99
00-01

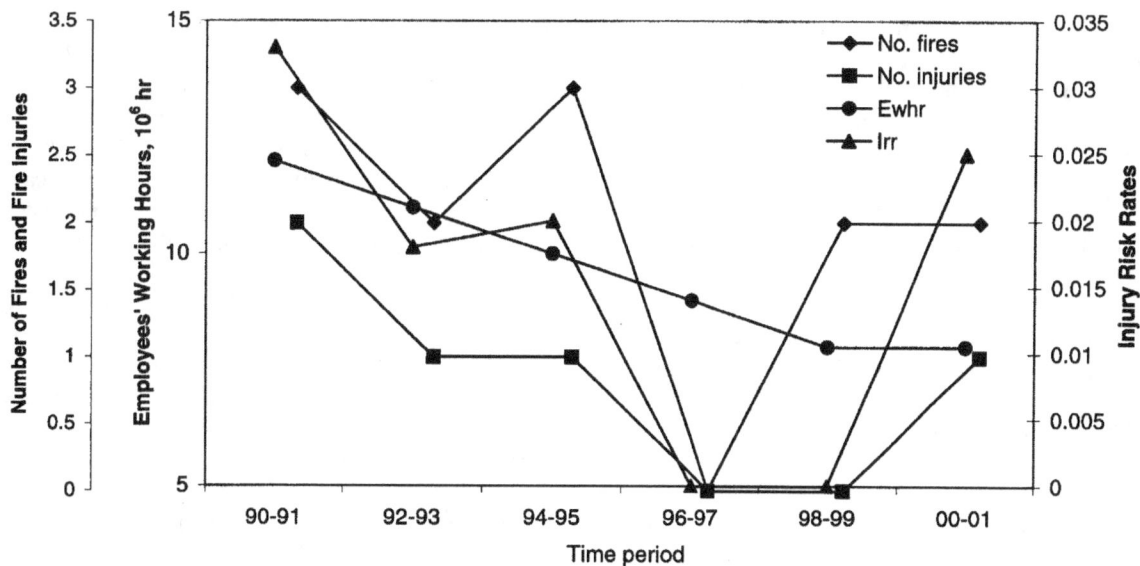

Figure 5.—Number of fires, fire injuries, risk rates, and employees' working hours for surface of underground metal/nonmetal and stone mines by time period, 1990–2001.

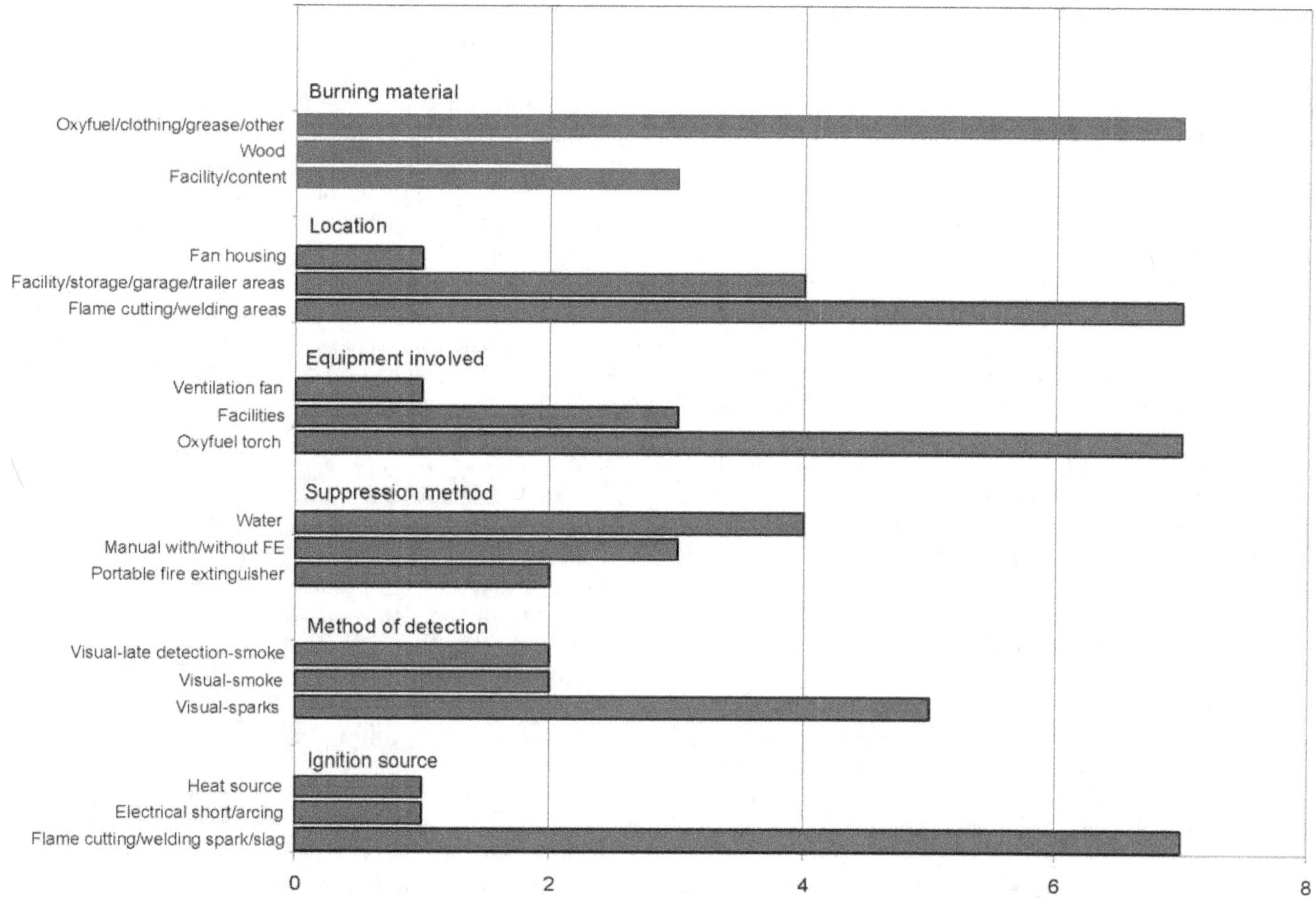

Burning material
Oxyfuel/clothing/grease/other
Wood
Facility/content
Location
Fan housing
Facility/storage/garage/trailer areas
Flame cutting/welding areas
Equipment involved
Ventilation fan
Facilities
Oxyfuel torch
Suppression method
Water
Manual with/without FE
Portable fire extinguisher
Method of detection
Visual-late detection-smoke
Visual-smoke
Visual-sparks
Ignition source
Heat source
Electrical short/arcing
Flame cutting/welding spark/slag

Figure 6.—Major variables for surface of underground metal/nonmetal and stone mine fires, 1990–2001. (FE = portable fire extinguisher)

Suppression Method

Table 14 shows the number of fires by suppression method for each time period. The most common method was water alone, followed by manual techniques with or without portable fire extinguishers and portable fire extinguishers alone. In three instances the fires destroyed or heavily damaged facilities because of failure of firefighting methods, undetected fire, or fire size.

During the first period, the largest number of fires were suppressed manually with or without portable fire extinguishers. During subsequent periods, the fires were extinguished with portable fire extinguishers alone (second period), water alone (third and fifth periods), and portable fire extinguishers or water alone (sixth period).

Equipment Involved

Table 15 shows the number of fires by equipment involved for each time period. The equipment most often involved was oxyfuel torches (at times electrical arc welding equipment was used), followed by facilities (considered equipment in this report), a heater, and a ventilation fan.

During the first and third periods, the largest number of fires involved oxyfuel torches. During the other periods, the fires involved oxyfuel torches and facilities (second period), facilities and a heater (fifth period), and an oxyfuel torch and a ventilation fan (sixth period).

Location

Table 16 shows the number of fires by location for each time period. The most common locations were flame cutting/welding areas (at shops, junction boxes, facilities, handrails, head frames, walkways, and maintenance areas), followed by facilities, garages, trailers and storage areas, and a ventilation fan housing.

During the first and third periods, the largest number of fires occurred at the flame cutting/welding areas. During the other periods, the fires occurred at flame cutting/welding areas and at facility, garage, trailer, and storage areas (second period), facilities (fifth period), and flame cutting/welding areas and fan housing (sixth period).

Burning Materials

Table 17 shows the number of fires by burning material for each time period. The materials most often involved were oxyfuel/clothing/grease and other materials (including electrical junction boxes, handrails, rubber tires, flammable liquids, and equipment mechanical components). Other burning materials involved facilities and their contents, and wood.

During the first and third periods, the largest number of fires involved oxyfuel, clothing, grease, and other materials. During the other periods, the fires involved oxyfuel and facilities and their contents (second period), wood and facilities (fifth period), and oxyfuel and wood (sixth period).

Fire Injuries

Table 18 shows the number of fire injuries per number of fires causing injuries and total fires by year, ignition source, equipment involved, and location during 1990–2001. In 1990, 1991, 1993, 1994, and 2000, there was one injury caused by one fire for each year. The cause of these fires was the flame cutting/welding spark/slag/flame ignition source.

SURFACE METAL/NONMETAL MINE FIRES

Table 19 and figure 7 show the number of fires and fire injuries for surface metal/nonmetal mines by state during 1990–2001. Table 19 also shows the injury risk rates, employees' working hours, and lost workdays. A total of 79 fires occurred in 16 states during 1990–2001 for these mines.

Forty-five of the fires caused 44 injuries and 2 fatalities (including 9 fires and 7 injuries involving contractors). The yearly average was 6.6 fires and 3.7 injuries. Sixty-five fires with 31 injuries and 2 fatalities occurred at metal mines, and 14 fires with 13 injuries occurred at nonmetal mines. The Ewhr value was 546×10^6 hr (Irr = 0.016), and the LWD value was 13,134.

Nevada and Arizona had the most fires (19 fires, 10 injuries, and 1 fatality; and 19 fires and 11 injuries, respectively). They were followed by Minnesota (11 fires, 4 injuries, and 1 fatality) and Alaska (6 fires and 4 injuries). Of these states, Alaska had the highest injury risk rate value (Irr = 0.079).

Table 20, partly illustrated in figure 8, shows the number of fires, fire injuries, fire fatalities, risk rates, employees' working hours, and lost workdays by time period. The number of fires increased during the second period, then decreased during most of the remaining periods. The number of fire injuries decreased during most of the periods (a small increase is seen during the last period), accompanied by a decline in employees' working hours during most of the periods (a small increase is seen during the third and fourth periods). The Irr values follow patterns similar to those shown by the number of fire injuries.

Tables 21–26 show the number of fires by ignition source, method of detection and suppression, equipment involved, location, and burning material by time period. Figure 9 shows the major variables related to fires for 1990–2001. Table 27 shows the number of fire injuries per number of fires causing injuries and total fires by year, ignition source, equipment involved, and location.

Ignition Source

Table 21 shows the number of fires and fire injuries by ignition source for each time period. The leading source was hydraulic fluid/fuel sprayed onto equipment hot surfaces (35 fires or 44%), followed by flame cutting/welding spark/slag/flame (13 fires or 17%) and electrical short/arcing (8 fires or 10%). Other sources were heat source-flammable liquid/vapors, flammable liquid/combustible material/refueling fuel on hot surfaces, overheated oil, hot material, and conveyor belt friction. Three ignition sources were unknown. Twenty-two of the 35 equipment hydraulic/fuel fires became large fires because of continuous flow of fluids from the pumps due to engine shutoff failure, difficulty in activating available emergency systems at ground level, lack of an emergency line drainage system, or lack of effective and rapid local firefighting response capabilities. In at least five instances, the cab was suddenly engulfed in flames, probably due to the ignition of flammable vapors and mists that penetrated the cab. Of note is that the hydraulic fluid fires subsequently involved the fuel system.

During the first through fourth and the sixth periods, the largest number of fires were caused by hydraulic fluid/fuel sprayed onto equipment hot surfaces. During the fifth period, the largest number of fires were caused by flame cutting/welding spark/slag/flame.

Table 19.—Number of fires, fire injuries, fire fatalities, and risk rates for surface metal/nonmetal mines by state, employees' working hours, and lost workdays, 1990–2001

State[1]	No. fires[1]	No. fire injuries[1]	LWD[2]	Ewhr,[2] 10^6 hr	Irr[3]
Alabama	1	1	—	1.6	0.125
Alaska	6	4	72	10.1	0.079
Arizona	19	11	243	88.4	0.025
California	5	1	—	25.7	0.008
Florida	3	3	52	42.4	0.014
Georgia	3	4	17.6	15.4	0.052
Idaho	2	1	—	7.7	0.026
Michigan	1	—	—	7.3	—
Minnesota[4]	11	4	6,236	12.3	0.065
Missouri	2	1	—	1	0.2
Nevada[4]	19	10	6,419	109	0.018
New Mexico	2	—	—	21.2	—
North Carolina	2	2	46	10.2	0.039
South Carolina	1	1	36	2	0.1
Texas	1	1	12	6.4	0.031
Wyoming	1	—	—	4.5	—
All other states	—	—	—	181	—
Total	79	44	13,134	546	[3]0.016

[1]Derived from MSHA "Fire Accident Abstract" internal publications.
[2]Derived from MSHA "Injury Experience in Mining" publications.
[3]Calculated according to MSHA formula reported in the "Methodologies" section.
[4]Minnesota and Nevada each had a fire fatality. These were caused by hydraulic fluid/fuel fires involving a dozer and a truck, respectively.

Table 20.—Number of fires, fire injuries, fire fatalities, and risk rates for surface metal/nonmetal mines by time period, employees' working hours, and lost workdays, 1990–2001

	Time period						
	90-91	92-93	94-95	96-97	98-99	00-01	1990-2001
Number of fires[1]	16	22	15	13	6	7	79
Number of fire injuries[1]	11	10	8	5	4	6	44
Number of fatalities[1]	—	—	1	—	—	1	2
LWD[2]	224	281	6,109	132	44	6,344	13,134
Ewhr,[2] 10^6 hr	97	93	95	98	83	80	546
Irr[3]	0.023	0.021	0.017	0.01	0.01	0.015	[3]0.016

[1]Derived from MSHA "Fire Accident Abstract" internal publications.
[2]Derived from MSHA "Injury Experience in Mining" publications.
[3]Calculated according to MSHA formula reported in the "Methodologies" section.

Table 21.—Number of fires for surface metal/nonmetal mines by ignition source and time period, 1990–2001

Ignition source	Time period						
	90-91 No. fires	92-93 No. fires	94-95 No. fires	96-97 No. fires	98-99 No. fires	00-01 No. fires	1990-2001 No. fires
Hydraulic fluid/fuel/oil on equipment hot surfaces	7	11	6	8	—	3	35
Flame cutting/welding spark/slag/flame	3	4	2	—	2	2	13
Electrical short/arcing	2	2	2	1	—	1	8
Heat source-flammable liquid/vapors	1	1	2	1	1	1	7
Flammable liquid/combustible material/refueling fuel on hot surfaces	2	2	2	—	1	—	7
Overheated oil	1	1	—	—	—	—	2
Hot material	—	—	—	1	1	—	2
Conveyor belt/equipment friction	—	—	1	1	—	—	2
Unknown/other	—	1	—	1	1	—	3
Total	16	22	15	13	6	7	79

Table 22.—Number of fires for surface metal/nonmetal mines by method of detection and time period, 1990–2001

Method of detection	Time period						
	90-91 No. fires	92-93 No. fires	94-95 No. fires	96-97 No. fires	98-99 No. fires	00-01 No. fires	1990-2001 No. fires
Visual:							
Flames/flash fires	6	11	8	7	1	4	37
Smoke	5	4	4	4	1	2	20
Sparks	3	3	2	—	2	1	11
Late smoke detection	2	2	1	2	1	—	8
Undetected	—	2	—	—	1	—	3
Total	16	22	15	13	6	7	79

Table 23.—Number of fires for surface metal/nonmetal mines by suppression method and time period, 1990–2001

Suppression method	Time period						
	90-91 No. fires	92-93 No. fires	94-95 No. fires	96-97 No. fires	98-99 No. fires	00-01 No. fires	1990-2001 No. fires
FE-foam-DCP-water	3	5	6	9	—	3	26
FE	6	5	5	1	3	2	22
Manual with or without FE[1]	3	3	2	1	1	1	11
Water	2	2	—	1	1	1	7
FSS-DCP-water	1	1	2	—	—	—	4
FSS-HD[2]	1	—	—	—	—	—	1
Destroyed/HD[3]	—	6	—	1	1	—	8
Total	16	22	15	13	6	7	79

DCP   Dry chemical powder.
FE   Portable fire extinguisher.
FSS   Machine fire suppression system.
HD   Heavily damaged.
[1]Method used by welders to extinguish clothing and oxyfuel/grease fires.
[2]Heavy damage to equipment due to FSS activation failure.
[3]Usually due to failure of firefighting methods, late fire detection, undetected fires, or fire size.

Table 24.—Number of fires for surface metal/nonmetal mines by equipment involved and time period, 1990–2001

Equipment	Time period						
	90-91 No. fires	92-93 No. fires	94-95 No. fires	96-97 No. fires	98-99 No. fires	00-01 No. fires	1990-2001 No. fires
Mobile equipment[1]	9	14	10	10	1	3	47
Oxyfuel torch[2]	3	4	2	—	2	2	13
Heater	2	1	1	—	1	2	7
Maintenance equipment	1	1	1	—	—	—	3
Generator	1	—	1	—	—	—	2
Facility[3]	—	1	—	—	1	—	2
Beltline	—	—	—	1	—	—	1
Chute	—	—	—	—	1	—	1
Sump	—	1	—	—	—	—	1
Other	—	—	—	2	—	—	2
Total	16	22	15	13	6	7	79

[1]Includes loaders, dozers, trucks, shovels, drills, and scrapers.
[2]At times, electrical arc welding equipment was used.
[3]Considered equipment in this report.

Table 25.—Number of fires for surface metal/nonmetal mines by location and time period, 1990–2001

Location	Time period						
	90-91 No. fires	92-93 No. fires	94-95 No. fires	96-97 No. fires	98-99 No. fires	00-01 No. fires	1990-2001 No. fires
Mobile equipment working areas[1]	8	13	10	10	—	3	44
Flame cutting/welding areas[2]	3	4	2	—	2	2	13
Maintenance/storage/refuse areas	3	3	2	—	3	1	12
Facility/shop/roofing areas	2	—	—	—	1	1	4
Generator housing/crusher/fire training areas ...	—	—	1	2	—	—	3
Waste dump/sump areas	—	2	—	1	—	—	3
Total	16	22	15	13	6	7	79

[1]Includes mining, haulage, drilling, loading, and excavating areas.
[2]Includes pipeline, dump rope, crowd platform, and maintenance areas.

Table 26.—Number of fires for surface metal/nonmetal mines by burning material and time period, 1990–2001

Burning material	Time period						
	90-91 No. fires	92-93 No. fires	94-95 No. fires	96-97 No. fires	98-99 No. fires	00-01 No. fires	1990-2001 No. fires
Hydraulic fluid/fuel/oil	7	11	5	8	—	3	34
Oxyfuel/clothing/grease/other[1]	3	4	2	—	2	2	13
Flammable liquid/combustible material ...	2	2	3	1	2	1	11
Electrical wires/cables	2	2	2	1	—	1	8
Refuse/wood/tires/chute liner	1	1	—	2	1	—	5
Equipment mechanical components	1	1	2	—	—	—	4
Facility/content	—	1	—	—	1	—	2
Belt material	—	—	1	1	—	—	2
Total	16	22	15	13	6	7	79

[1]Includes rubber hoses, pipeline, dump rope cables, grease, screen liner, shaft material, and equipment mechanical components.

Table 27.—Number of fire injuries per number of fires causing injuries and total fires for surface metal/nonmetal mines by year, ignition source, equipment involved, and location, 1990–2001

Year	No. total fires	No. fires causing injuries	No. fire injuries	Ignition source	Equipment	Location
1990	5	3	1	Flame cutting/welding spark/slag/flame	Oxyfuel torch	Flame cutting/welding areas.
			1	Hydraulic fluid/fuel on equipment hot surfaces	Truck	Haulage area.
			1	Oil on hot surfaces	Truck	Haulage area.
1991	11	7	2	Flame cutting/welding spark/slag/flame	Oxyfuel torch	Flame cutting/welding areas.
			1	Flammable liquid on hot surfaces	Maintenance equipment	Refuse pile area.
			5	Hydraulic fluid/fuel on equipment hot surfaces	Loader/truck/dozer	Loading/haulage/mining areas.
1992	13	5	2	Flame cutting/welding spark/slag/flame	Oxyfuel torch	Flame cutting/welding areas.
			1	Flammable liquid on hot surfaces	Maintenance equipment	Maintenance area.
			1	Heat source-flammable vapors	Heater	Maintenance area.
			1	Hydraulic fluid/fuel on equipment hot surfaces	Loader	Loading area.
1993	9	5	1	Flame cutting/welding spark/slag/flame	Oxyfuel torch	Flame cutting/welding areas.
			1	Refueling fuel on hot surfaces	Truck	Maintenance area.
			2	Hydraulic fluid/fuel on equipment hot surfaces	Scraper/loader	Mining/loading areas.
			1	Electrical short/arcing	Truck	Haulage area.
1994	10	4	1	Flame cutting/welding spark/slag/flame	Oxyfuel torch	Flame cutting/welding areas.
			1	Electrical short/arcing	Generator	Generator housing.
			1	Heat source	Heater	Maintenance area.
			1	Hydraulic fluid/fuel on equipment hot surfaces	Truck	Haulage area.
1995[1] ...	5	5	1	Flame cutting/welding spark/slag/flame	Oxyfuel torch	Flame cutting/welding areas.
			1	Flammable liquid on hot surfaces	Maintenance equipment	Storage facility.
			2	Hydraulic fluid/fuel on equipment hot surfaces	Truck	Haulage area.
1996	6	4	3	Hydraulic fluid/fuel on equipment hot surfaces	Truck	Haulage area.
			1	Oil on hot surfaces	Truck	Dump area.
1997	7	1	1	Heat source-flammable liquid	Matches	Fire training facility.
1998	1	1	1	Flame cutting/welding spark/slag/flame	Oxyfuel torch	Flame cutting/welding areas.
1999	5	3	1	Heat source	Heater	Maintenance areas.
			1	Flammable liquid on hot surfaces	Truck	Maintenance areas.
			1	Flame cutting/welding spark/slag/flame	Oxyfuel torch	Flame cutting/welding areas.
2000[1] ...	5	5	1	Heat source	Heater	Maintenance area.
			2	Hydraulic fluid/fuel on equipment hot surfaces	Truck	Haulage area.
			1	Flame cutting/welding spark/slag/flame	Oxyfuel torch	Flame cutting/welding areas.
2001	2	2	2	Flame cutting/welding spark/slag/flame	Oxyfuel torch	Flame cutting/welding areas.
Total	79	45	44			

[1]A fire fatality occurred in 1995 and 2000. These were caused by hydraulic fluid/fuel fires involving a truck and a dozer, respectively.

Method of Detection

Table 22 shows the number of fires by method of detection for each time period. The most frequent methods were operators who saw the fires when they started as flames/flash fires, miners who saw smoke shortly after the fires had started, and welders who saw sparks. Other methods of detection were miners who saw smoke long after the fires had started. Three fires were undetected. During the first through fourth and the sixth periods, the largest number of fires were detected by operators as flames/flash fires. During the fifth period, the largest number of fires were detected by welders as sparks.

Suppression Method

Table 23 shows the number of fires by suppression method for each time period. The most common methods were portable fire extinguishers with foam, dry chemical powder, and water, followed by portable fire extinguishers alone and manual techniques with or without portable fire extinguishers. Other methods were water alone and machine fire suppression systems with dry chemical powder, foam, and water. Five of the 35 pieces of mobile equipment involved in the hydraulic fluid/ fuel fires had machine fire suppression systems. Dual activation (one activaion) of machine fire suppression and engine shutoff systems succeeded in temporarily abating the fires; however, the flames reignited, fueled by the flow of pressurized fluids entrapped in the lines. On three other occasions (one of which resulted in a fatality), the fires raged out of control because of machine fire suppression system failure. In another instance the fire was detected late.

On at least five occasions, including one mobile equipment fire, fire brigades and fire departments fought the fires with foam, dry chemical powder, and water. However, eight fires destroyed or heavily damaged equipment (including seven pieces of mobile equipment) because of failure of firefighting methods, late fire detection, undetected fires, or fire size.

During the first and fifth periods, the largest number of fires were suppressed with portable fire extinguishers alone. During the second period, the largest number of fires were suppressed with portable fire extinguishers together with foam, dry chemical powder, and water and with portable fire extinguishers alone. During the third, fourth, and sixth periods, the largest number of fires were suppressed with portable fire extinguishers, foam, dry chemical powder, and water.

Equipment Involved

Table 24 shows the number of fires by equipment involved for each time period. The equipment most often involved was mobile equipment (trucks, dozers, loaders, shovels, drills, and scrapers), followed by oxyfuel torches (at times electrical arc welding equipment was used) and heaters. Other equipment included maintenance equipment, beltlines, generators, chutes, a sump, and facilities (considered equipment in this report). During the first through fourth and the sixth periods, the largest number of fires involved mobile equipment. During the fifth period, the largest number of fires involved oxyfuel torches.

Table 28.—Number of fires, fire injuries, and risk rates for surface sand and gravel mines by state, employees' working hours, and lost workdays, 1990–2001

State[1]	No. fires[1]	No. fire injuries[1]	LWD[2]	Ewhr,[2] 10^6 hr	Irr[3]
Arizona	3	3	63	15	0.04
Arkansas	1	1	—	10	0.02
California	9	5	160	89.4	0.011
Colorado	2	2	6	24	0.017
Florida	2	2	—	15	0.027
Illinois	3	3	54	20.7	0.029
Indiana	2	2	22	21.3	0.019
Kansas	1	1	—	8	0.025
Kentucky	1	1	7	6	0.033
Louisiana	4	4	29	15	0.053
Maryland	1	1	3	11.2	0.018
Michigan	6	6	69	33.5	0.036
Mississippi	3	3	54	6.3	0.095
Missouri	1	1	32	10	0.02
Nebraska	2	2	34	11	0.036
New Hampshire	2	2	8	26.5	0.015
New York	3	2	16	28	0.014
Ohio	4	2	65	37	0.011
Oklahoma	1	—	—	10	—
Oregon	1	1	16	13.7	0.015
Pennsylvania	5	5	76	19.3	0.052
South Carolina	1	—	—	10.2	—
South Dakota	2	2	35	5.8	0.069
Texas	1	1	30	60	0.003
Utah	3	3	6,075	15.6	0.039
Virginia	1	—	—	10.4	—
Washington	1	1	20	25	0.008
Wisconsin	2	2	39	22	0.018
Wyoming	2	2	8	4.4	0.091
All other states	—	—	—	157	—
Total	70	60	6,921	741	[3]0.016

[1]Derived from MSHA "Fire Accident Abstract" internal publications.
[2]Derived from MSHA "Injury Experience in Mining" publications.
[3]Calculated according to MSHA formula reported in the "Methodologies" section.

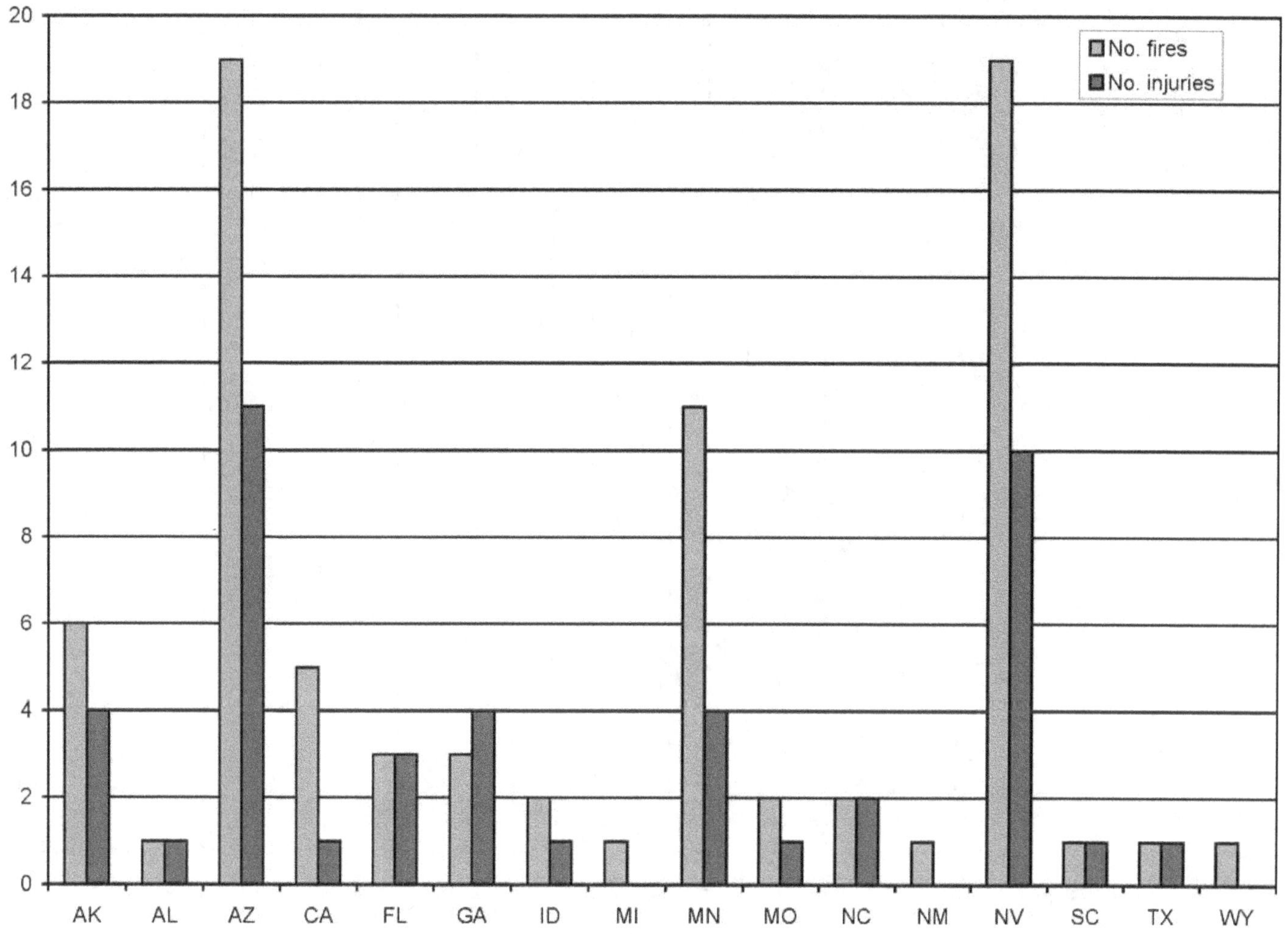

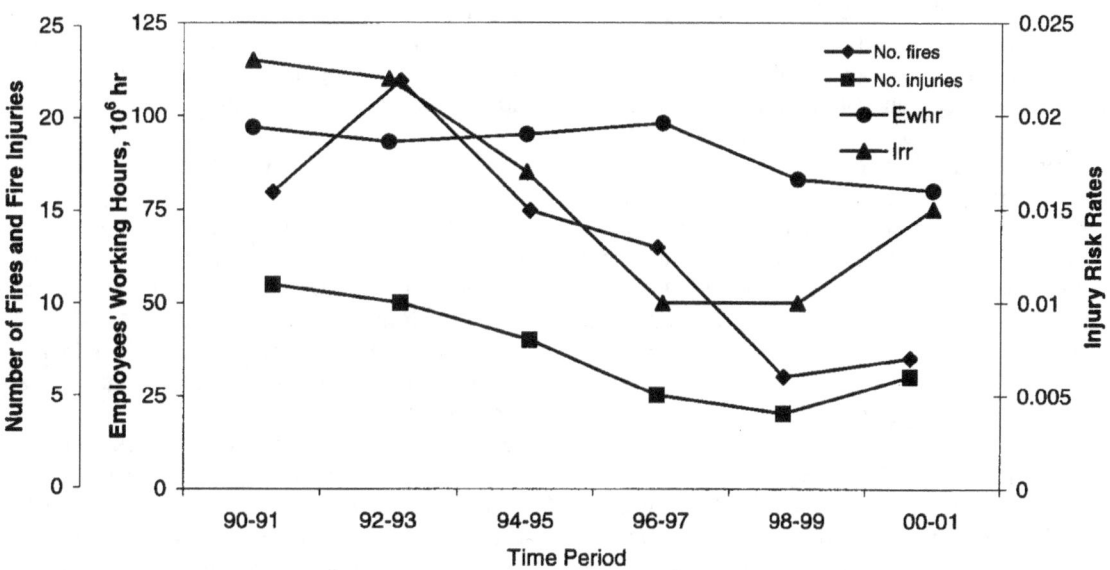

Figure 7.—Number of fires and fire injuries for surface metal/nonmetal mines by state, 1990–2001.

Figure 8.—Number of fires, fire injuries, risk rates, and employees' working hours for surface metal/nonmetal mines by time period, 1990–2001.

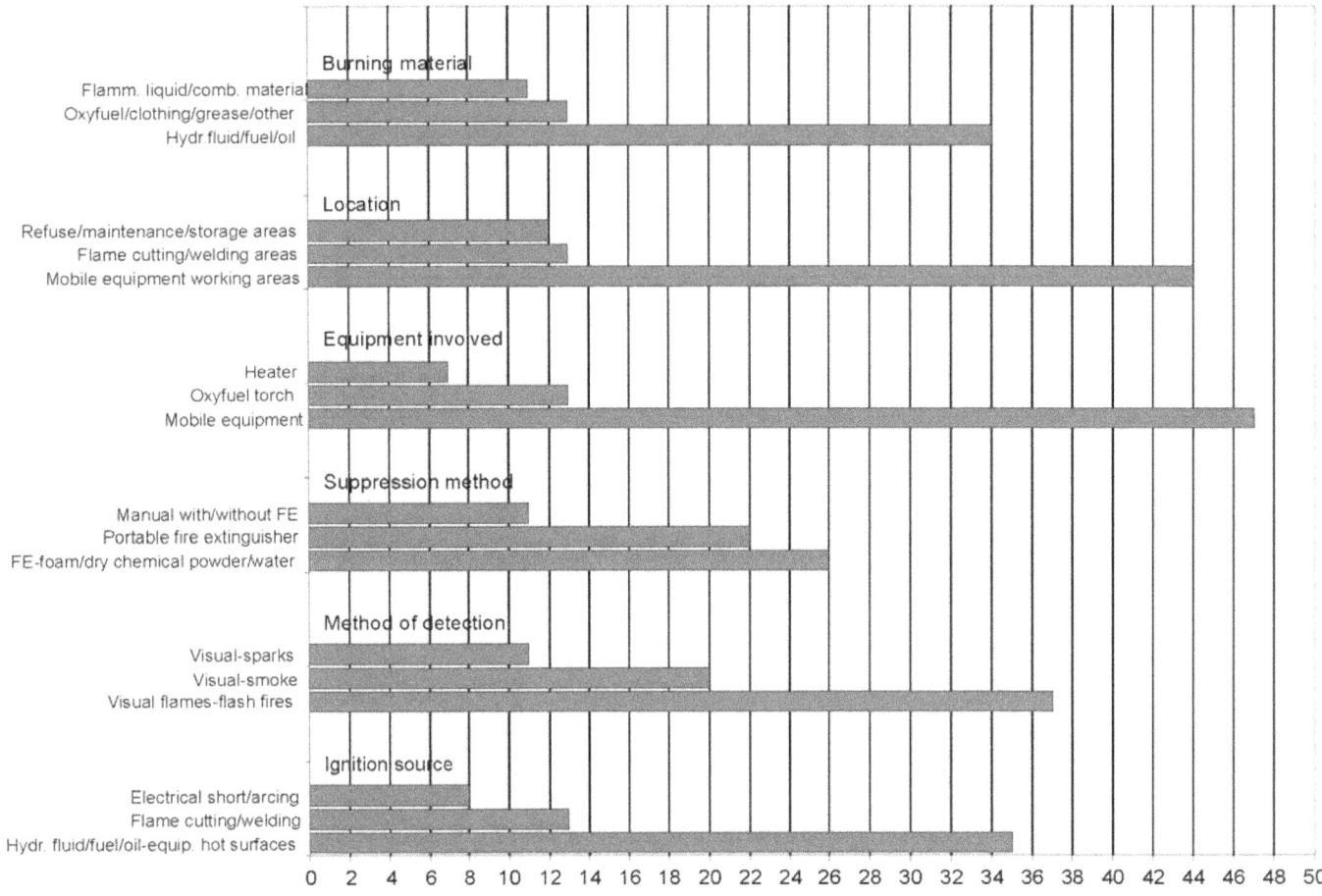

Figure 9.—Major variables for surface metal/nonmetal mine fires, 1990–2001. (FE = portable fire extinguisher)

Location

Table 25 shows the number of fires by location for each time period. The most common locations were mobile equipment working areas (mining, haulage, loading, drilling, and excavating areas). This was followed by flame cutting/welding areas (at pipeline, dump rope, crowd platform, and maintenance areas) and maintenance, storage, and refuse areas. Other fire locations included facilities and roofing areas, waste dump and sump areas, and generator housing, crusher, and fire training areas. During the first through fourth and the sixth periods, the largest number of fires occurred at mobile equipment working areas. During the fifth period, the largest number of fires occurred at maintenance, storage, and refuse areas.

Burning Materials

Table 26 shows the number of fires by burning material for each time period. The material most often involved was hydraulic fluid/fuel, followed by oxyfuel/clothing/grease and other materials (including rubber hoses, pipelines, grease, equipment mechanical components, dump rope cables, screen liner, and shaft material), flammable liquids, and combustible materials. Other burning materials involved electrical wires and cables, refuse, wood, tires and chute liner, equipment mechanical components, facilities and their content, and belt material. During the first through fourth and the sixth periods, the largest number of fires involved hydraulic fluid/fuel and oil. During the fifth period, the largest number of fires involved oxyfuel, flammable liquids, and combustible materials.

Fire Injuries

Table 27 shows the number of fire injuries per number of fires causing injuries and total fires by year, ignition source, equipment involved, and location for 1990–2001. Overall, there were 44 injuries and 2 fatalities caused by 45 fires. The greatest number of fire injuries occurred in 1991 (eight injuries caused by seven fires). The ignition sources that caused most of the fire injuries were hydraulic fluid/fuel sprayed onto equipment hot surfaces and flame cutting/welding spark/slag/flame. Other ignition sources causing injuries were flammable liquid/refueling fuel on hot surfaces, heat source-vapors/flammable liquid, electrical short/arcing, and oil on hot surfaces. The equipment most often involved in fire injuries included mobile equipment, oxyfuel torches, and maintenance equipment, followed by heaters, electrical systems, and air compressors. The locations where the fire injuries occurred were mobile equipment working areas, flame cutting/welding areas, maintenance and fire training areas, and generator housing.

Nevada and Minnesota each had a fire fatality [MSHA 1995e, 2000e]. These were caused by hydraulic fluid/fuel fires involving a truck and a dozer, respectively. The victims were severely burned while exiting the cab.

SURFACE SAND AND GRAVEL MINE FIRES

Table 28 and figure 10 show the number of fires and fire injuries for surface sand and gravel mines by state during 1990–2001. Table 28 also shows the injury risk rates, employees' working hours, and lost workdays. At surface sand and gravel mines, a total of 70 fires with 60 injuries occurred in 29 states during 1990–2001. Fifty-nine of the fires caused 60 injuries (none of the fires involved contractors). The yearly average was 5.8 fires and five injuries. The Ewhr value was 741×10^6 hr (Irr = 0.016), and the LWD value was 6,921. California had the most fires (nine fires and five injuries), followed by Michigan (six fires and six injuries) and Pennsylvania (five fires and five injuries). Of these states, Pennsylvania had the highest injury risk rate value (Irr = 0.052).

Table 29, partly illustrated in figure 11, shows the number of fires, fire injuries, risk rates, employees' working hours, and lost workdays by time period. The number of fires and fire injuries show an increase during the second period followed by a decrease during the fourth period followed by a small increase during the fifth period and a sharp decrease during the last period. Employees' working hours increased during most of the periods. The Irr values follow patterns similar to those shown by the injury values.

Tables 30–35 show the number of fires by ignition source, method of detection and suppression, equipment involved, location, and burning material by time period. Figure 12 shows the major variables related to fires for 1990–2001. Table 36 shows the fire injuries per number of fires causing injuries and total fires by year, ignition source, equipment involved, and location.

Ignition Source

Table 30 shows the number of fires by ignition source for each time period. The leading source was flame cutting/welding spark/slag/flame (29 fires or 41%), followed by heat source/explosion (15 fires or 21%) involving pressurized cans and flammable liquids and by hydraulic fluid/fuel sprayed onto equipment hot surfaces (14 fires or 20%). Other ignition sources were flammable liquid/gas/refueling fuel on hot surfaces/collision (in one instance, the fuel ignited upon equipment collision) and electrical short/arcing/explosion (involving a pump). Two ignition sources were unknown. At least 5 of the 14 mobile equipment hydraulic fluid/fuel fires became large fires because of the continuous flow of fluids from the pumps due to engine shutoff failure, difficulty in activating available emergency systems at ground level, lack of an emergency drainage system, or lack of effective and rapid local firefighting response capabilities. On two occasions, the cab was suddenly engulfed in flames, probably due to the ignition of flammable vapors and mists that penetrated the cab. Of note is that the hydraulic fluid fires subsequently involved the fuel system. During all of the periods, the largest number of fires were caused by flame cutting/welding spark/slag/flame.

Table 29.—Number of fires, fire injuries, and risk rates for surface sand and gravel mines by time period, employees' working hours, and lost workdays, 1990–2001

	Time period						
	90-91	92-93	94-95	96-97	98-99	00-01	1990-2001
Number of fires[1]	8	16	16	11	13	6	70
Number of fire injuries[1]	7	13	15	8	11	6	60
LWD[2]	73	193	218	6,089	234	114	6,921
Ewhr,[2] 10^6 hr	115	112	118	122	134	140	741
Irr[3]	0.012	0.023	0.025	0.013	0.016	0.009	[3]0.016

[1]Derived from MSHA "Fire Accident Abstract" internal publications.
[2]Derived from MSHA "Injury Experience in Mining" publications.
[3]Calculated according to MSHA formula reported in the "Methodologies" section.

Table 30.—Number of fires for surface sand and gravel mines by ignition source and time period, 1990–2001

Ignition source	Time period						
	90-91 No. fires	92-93 No. fires	94-95 No. fires	96-97 No. fires	98-99 No. fires	00-01 No. fires	1990-2001 No. fires
Flame cutting/welding spark/slag/flame	4	6	6	5	5	3	29
Heat source/explosion[1]	2	3	5	2	1	2	15
Hydraulic fluid/fuel on equipment hot surfaces	—	5	4	2	2	1	14
Flammable liquid/gas/refueling fuel on hot surfaces/ equipment collision	2	2	—	1	1	—	6
Electrical short/arcing/explosion[2]	—	—	1	1	2	—	4
Unknown	—	—	—	—	2	—	2
Total	8	16	16	11	13	6	70

[1]Involving pressurized cans and flammable liquid.
[2]Involving a pump.

Table 31.—Number of fires for surface sand and gravel mines by method of detection and time period,
1990–2001

Method of detection	Time period						
	90-91 No. fires	92-93 No. fires	94-95 No. fires	96-97 No. fires	98-99 No. fires	00-01 No. fires	1990-2001 No. fires
Visual:							
Flames/flash fires	2	5	3	3	4	4	21
Sparks	4	5	6	1	4	1	21
Smoke	—	3	4	3	—	1	11
Late smoke detection	1	2	—	3	2	—	8
Heard an explosion	1	—	2	—	1	—	4
Power loss	—	1	—	—	—	—	1
Undetected	—	—	1	1	2	—	4
Total	8	16	16	11	13	6	70

Table 32.—Number of fires for surface sand and gravel mines by suppression method and time period,
1990–2001

Suppression method	Time period						
	90-91 No. fires	92-93 No. fires	94-95 No. fires	96-97 No. fires	98-99 No. fires	00-01 No. fires	1990-2001 No. fires
Manual with or without FE[1]	4	5	6	2	4	3	24
FE-DCP-foam-water	1	6	4	4	4	1	20
Water	1	4	5	3	1	2	16
FE	2	1	—	1	2	—	6
Destroyed/HD[2]	—	—	1	1	2	—	4
Total	8	16	16	11	13	6	70

DCP Dry chemical powder.
FE Portable fire extinguisher.
HD Heavily damaged.
[1]Method used by welders to extinguish clothing and oxyfuel/grease fires.
[2]Usually due to failure of firefighting methods, late fire detection, undetected fires, or fire size.

Table 33.—Number of fires for surface sand and gravel mines by equipment involved and time period,
1990–2001

Equipment	Time period						
	90-91 No. fires	92-93 No. fires	94-95 No. fires	96-97 No. fires	98-99 No. fires	00-01 No. fires	1990-2001 No. fires
Oxyfuel torch[1]	4	6	6	5	5	3	29
Mobile equipment[2]	2	5	5	2	3	1	18
Heater/burner	2	3	5	2	1	2	15
Generator/pump	—	—	—	1	2	—	3
Maintenance equipment	—	2	—	1	—	—	3
Facility[3]	—	—	—	—	2	—	2
Total	8	16	16	11	13	6	70

[1]At times, electrical arc welding equipment was used.
[2]Includes trucks, loaders, scrapers, dredges, backhoes, and buckets.
[3]Considered equipment in this report.

Table 34.—Number of fires for surface sand and gravel mines by location and time period, 1990–2001

Location	90-91 No. fires	92-93 No. fires	94-95 No. fires	96-97 No. fires	98-99 No. fires	00-01 No. fires	1990-2001 No. fires
Flame cutting/welding areas[1]	4	6	6	5	5	3	29
Maintenance areas	3	4	5	3	1	1	17
Mobile equipment working areas[2]	—	5	4	3	3	1	16
Generator/pump/electrical control areas	—	—	1	—	2	—	3
Facility area	—	—	—	—	2	—	2
Crusher/refuse areas	1	—	—	—	—	1	2
Beltline area	—	1	—	—	—	—	1
Total	8	16	16	11	13	6	70

[1]Includes beltline, water pipelines, chute, crusher, hopper and compactor areas, washer plants, and maintenance areas.
[2]Includes haulage, loading, mining, and dredging areas.

Table 35.—Number of fires for surface sand and gravel mines by burning material and time period, 1990–2001

Burning material	90-91 No. fires	92-93 No. fires	94-95 No. fires	96-97 No. fires	98-99 No. fires	00-01 No. fires	1990-2001 No. fires
Oxyfuel/clothing/grease/other[1]	4	6	6	5	5	3	29
Hydraulic fluid/fuel	—	5	4	2	2	1	14
Refuse/rubber tires	1	2	4	1	—	1	9
Flammable liquid/gas/refueling fuel	2	2	1	2	1	1	9
Electrical control wires/cables	—	—	1	1	2	—	4
Belt material/crusher	1	1	—	—	1	—	3
Facility/content	—	—	—	—	2	—	2
Total	8	16	16	11	13	6	70

[1]Includes chute liner, washer plant, flammable liquids, shaker deck, belt material, crusher and hopper, and equipment mechanical components.

Table 36.—Number of fire injuries per number of fires causing injuries and total fires for surface sand and gravel mines by year, ignition source, equipment involved, and location, 1990–2001

Year	No. total fires	No. fires causing injuries	No. fire injuries	Ignition source	Equipment	Location
1990	4	3	1	Flame cutting/welding spark/slag/flame	Oxyfuel torch	Flame cutting/welding areas.
			2	Refueling fuel on hot surfaces	Truck	Maintenance area.
1991	4	4	3	Flame cutting/welding spark/slag/flame	Oxyfuel torch	Flame cutting/welding areas.
			1	Heat source	Heater	Refuse area.
1992	9	6	2	Flammable liquid on hot surfaces	Maintenance equipment	Maintenance area.
			1	Heat source	Heater	Maintenance area.
			1	Flame cutting/welding spark/slag/flame	Oxyfuel torch	Flame cutting/welding areas.
			2	Hydraulic fluid/fuel on equipment hot surfaces	Truck	Haulage area.
1993	7	7	4	Flame cutting/welding spark/slag/flame	Oxyfuel torch	Flame cutting/welding areas.
			1	Heat source	Heater	Beltline areas.
			2	Hydraulic fluid/fuel on equipment hot surfaces	Dredge-loader	Dredging/loading areas.
1994	8	7	3	Flame cutting/welding spark/slag/flame	Oxyfuel torch	Flame cutting/welding areas.
			3	Heat source-flammable liquid	Heater	Maintenance area.
			1	Electrical short/arcing	Electrical system	Electrical control area.
1995	8	8	3	Heat source	Heater	Maintenance area.
			3	Flame cutting/welding spark/slag/flame	Oxyfuel torch	Flame cutting/welding areas.
			2	Hydraulic fluid/fuel on equipment hot surfaces	Loader/scraper	Loading/mining areas.
1996	7	6	1	Flame cutting/welding spark/slag/flame	Oxyfuel torch	Flame cutting/welding areas.
			2	Heat source	Heater	Maintenance area.
			1	Flammable liquid on hot surfaces	Maintenance equipment	Maintenance area.
			1	Hydraulic fluid/fuel on equipment hot surfaces	Loader	Loading area.
			1	Electrical short/arcing	Loader cab	Loading area.
1997	4	2	2	Flame cutting/welding spark/slag/flame	Oxyfuel torch	Flame cutting/welding areas.
1998	10	9	4	Flame cutting/welding spark/slag/flame	Oxyfuel torch	Flame cutting/welding areas.
			3	Electrical short/arcing	Pump/generator	Pump/generator housing.
			1	Heat source	Heater	Maintenance area.
			2	Hydraulic fluid/fuel on equipment hot surfaces	Truck/loader	Haulage/loading areas.
1999	3	1	1	Flame cutting/welding spark/slag/flame	Oxyfuel torch	Flame cutting/welding areas.
2000	3	3	2	Heat source	Heater	Maintenance/refuse areas.
			1	Flame cutting/welding spark/slag/flame	Oxyfuel torch	Flame cutting/welding areas.
2001	3	3	2	Flame cutting/welding spark/slag/flame	Oxyfuel torch	Flame cutting/welding areas.
			1	Hydraulic fluid/fuel	Loader	Loading area.
Total	70	59	60			

Method of Detection

Table 31 shows the number of fires by method of detection for each time period. The most frequent methods were welders who saw sparks and operators who saw the fires when they started as flames/flash fires. Other methods of detection were miners who heard an explosion and operators who experienced an equipment power loss. Four fires were undetected.

During the first period, the largest number of fires were detected by welders as sparks. During the second and fifth periods, the largest number of fires were detected by operators and welders as flames/flash fires and sparks. During the third period, the largest number of fires were detected by welders as sparks. During the fourth period, the largest number of fires were detected by operators as flames/flash fires and by miners as smoke shortly or long after the fires had started. During the sixth period, the largest number of fires were detected by operators as flames/flash fires.

Suppression Method

Table 32 shows the number of fires by suppression method for each time period. The most frequent methods were manual techniques with or without portable fire extinguishers, portable

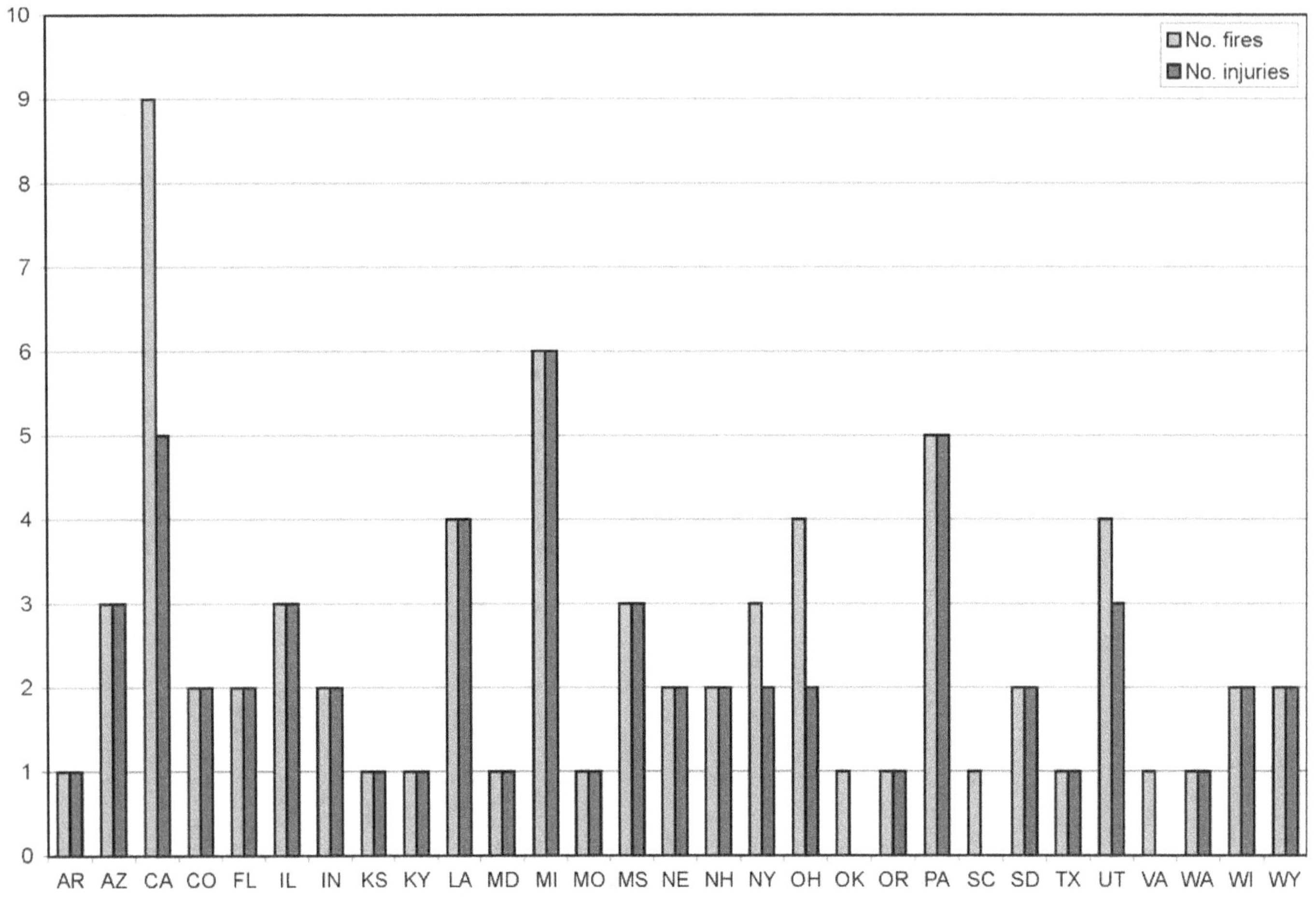

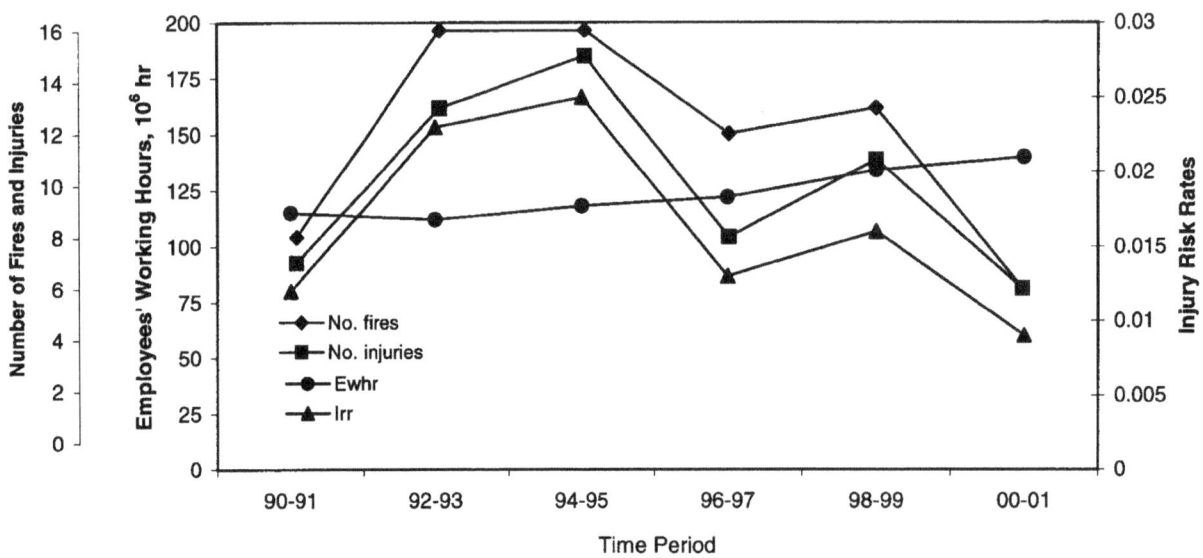

Figure 10.—Number of fires and fire injuries for surface sand and gravel mines by state, 1990–2001.

Figure 11.—Number of fires, fire injuries, risk rates, and employees' working hours for surface sand and gravel mines by time period, 1990–2001.

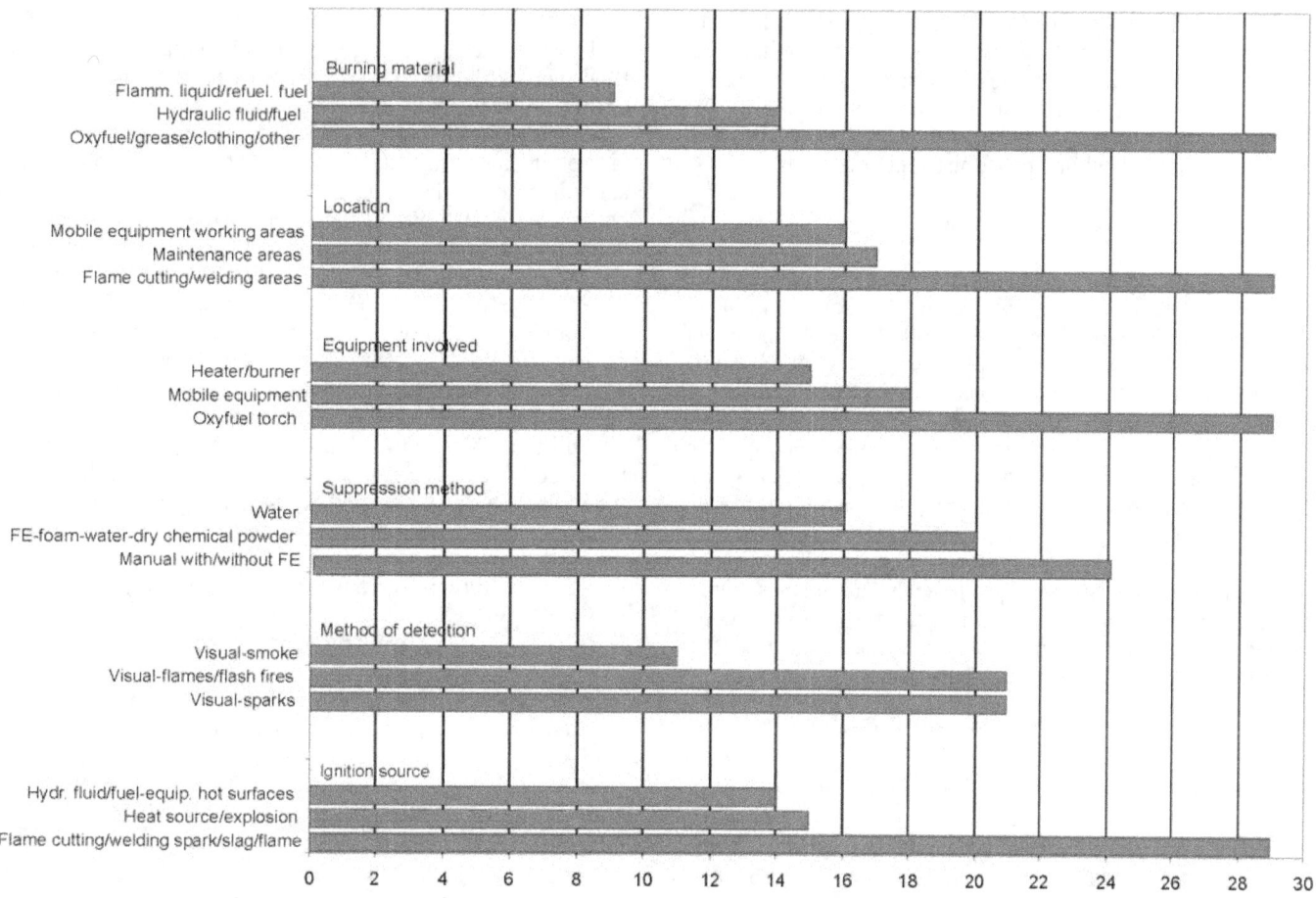

Figure 12.—Major variables for surface sand and gravel mine fires, 1990–2001. (FE = portable fire extinguisher)

fire extinguishers with dry chemical powder, foam and water, and water alone. Portable fire extinguishers alone were also used to suppress the fires. None of the equipment involved in fires had machine fire suppression systems. On at least three occasions, including one mobile equipment fire, fire brigades and fire departments fought the fires with foam, dry chemical powder, and water. However, in four instances the fires destroyed or heavily damaged equipment (including two pieces of mobile equipment) because of failure of other firefighting methods, late fire detection, undetected fires, or fire size.

During the first, third, and sixth periods, the largest number of fires were suppressed manually with or without portable fire extinguishers. During the second and fourth periods, the largest number of fires were suppressed with portable fire extinguishers together with dry chemical powder, foam, and water. During the fifth period, the largest number of fires were extinguished manually with or without portable fire extinguishers and with portable fire extinguishers, dry chemical powder, foam, and water.

Equipment Involved

Table 33 shows the number of fires by equipment involved for each time period. The equipment most often involved was oxyfuel torches (at times electrical arc welding equipment was used), followed by mobile equipment (loaders, trucks, scrapers, dredges,

backhoes, and buckets) and heaters/burners. Other equipment included maintenance equipment, generators and pumps, and facilities (considered equipment in this report). During all of the periods, the largest number of fires involved oxyfuel torches.

Location

Table 34 shows the number of fires by location for each time period. The most common locations were flame cutting/welding areas (at beltline, pipeline, chute, crusher, hopper, and compactor areas, washer plants, and maintenance areas), followed by maintenance areas and mobile equipment working areas (loading, haulage, mining, and dredging areas). Other fire locations included generator and pump housing, electrical control areas, facility areas, crusher and refuse areas, and beltline areas. During all of the periods, the largest number of fires occurred at flame cutting/welding areas.

Burning Materials

Table 35 shows the number of fires by burning material for each time period. The materials most often involved were oxyfuel/clothing/grease and other materials (including chute liner, washer plant, flammable liquids, equipment mechanical components, shaker deck, crusher and hopper, and belt material).

This was followed by hydraulic fluid/fuel and by flammable liquids, gas, and refueling fuel. Other burning materials included refuse and rubber tires, electrical control, wires and cables, belt material and crusher, and facilities and their contents. During all of the periods, the largest number of fires involved oxyfuel/clothing/grease and other materials.

Fire Injuries

Table 36 shows the number of fire injuries per number of fires causing injuries and total fires by year, ignition source, equipment involved, and location during 1990–2001. Overall, there were 60 injuries caused by 59 fires. The greatest number of fire injuries occurred in 1998 (10 injuries caused by 9 fires). The ignition sources that caused most of the fire injuries were flame cutting/welding spark/slag/flame, heat source, and hydraulic fluid/fuel sprayed onto equipment hot surfaces. Other ignition sources were flammable liquid/refueling fuel on hot surfaces and electrical short/arcing. The equipment most often involved in fire injuries included oxyfuel torches, heaters, and mobile equipment, followed by maintenance equipment, electrical systems, pumps, and generators. The locations where the fire injuries occurred were flame cutting/welding areas, maintenance areas, mobile equipment working areas, and pump and generator housing.

SURFACE STONE MINE FIRES

Table 37 and figure 13 show the number of fires and fire injuries for surface stone mines by state during 1990–2001. Table 37 also shows the injury risk rates, employees' working hours, and lost workdays. In all, 96 fires occurred in 31 states and 1 fire occurred in Puerto Rico. Sixty-eight of the fires caused 67 injuries and 1 fatality (including 6 fires and 5 injuries involving contractors). The yearly average was eight fires and 5.6 injuries. The Ewhr value was 689×10^6 hr (Irr = 0.02), and the LWD value was 7,399.

Indiana had the most fires (eight fires and four injuries), followed by Georgia (seven fires and seven injuries) and Pennsylvania (seven fires and five injuries). Of these states, Georgia had the highest injury risk rate value (Irr = 0.058).

Table 38, partly illustrated in figure 14, shows the number of fires, fire injuries, fire fatalities, risk rates, employees' working hours, and lost workdays by time period. The number of fires and fire injuries show an increase during the second period followed by a decrease during most of the remaining periods. Employees' working hours increased during most of the periods. The Irr values follow patterns similar to those shown by the injury values.

Tables 39–44 show the number of fires by ignition source, method of detection and suppression, equipment involved, location, and burning material by time period. Figure 15 shows the major variables related to fires for 1990–2001. Table 45 shows the number of fire injuries per number of fires causing injuries and total fires by year, ignition source, equipment involved, and location.

Ignition Source

Table 39 shows the number of fires and fire injuries by ignition source for each time period. The leading sources were flame cutting/welding spark/slag/flame (25 fires or 26%), heat source/explosion-flammable liquid (24 fires or 25%), and hy-draulic fluid/fuel sprayed onto equipment hot surfaces (16 fires or 17%). At least 10 of the 16 mobile equipment hydraulic fluid/fuel fires became large fires because of the continuous flow of fluids from the pumps due to engine shutoff failure, difficulty in activating available emergency systems at the ground level, lack of an emergency line drainage system, or lack of effective and rapid local firefighting response capabilities. On two occasions, the cab was suddenly engulfed in flames, probably due to the ignition of flammable vapors and mists that penetrated the cab. Of note is that the hydraulic fluid fires subsequently involved the fuel system. Other ignition sources were electrical short/arcing, refueling fuel/flammable liquid on hot surfaces, explosion/ignition of hazardous material, chemical and explosives, hot material, engine malfunction/mechanical friction, and overheated oil. Nine ignition sources were unknown.

During the first, third, fourth, and fifth periods, the largest number of fires were caused by heat source/explosion-flammable liquid/gas. During the second period, the largest number of fires were caused by flame cutting/welding spark/slag/flame. During the sixth period, the largest number of fires were caused by hydraulic fluid/fuel sprayed onto equipment hot surfaces.

Method of Detection

Table 40 shows the number of fires by method of detection for each time period. The most frequent methods were operators who saw the fires when they started as flames/flash fires, welders who saw sparks, and miners who saw smoke shortly after the fires had started. Other methods of detection were miners who heard an explosion or touched a hot spot, miners who saw smoke long after the fires had started, and operators who saw a white mist. Eight fires were undetected.

During the first period, the largest number of fires were detected by welders as sparks and by miners who heard an explosion. During the second period, the largest number of fires were detected by welders as sparks. During the third period, the largest number of fires were detected by operators as flames/flash fires and by welders as sparks. During the fourth and fifth periods, the largest number of fires were detected by miners as smoke. During the sixth period, the largest number of fires were detected by operators as flames/flash fires.

Suppression Method

Table 41 shows the number of fires by suppression method for each time period. The most common methods were manual techniques with or without portable fire extinguishers or water alone, portable fire extinguishers with dry chemical powder, and foam and water. None of the equipment involved in fires had machine fire suppression systems. On at least six occasions, including one mobile equipment fire, fire brigades and fire departments fought the fires with portable fire extinguishers, foam, dry chemical powder, and water. However, 12 fires destroyed or heavily damaged equipment (including four pieces of mobile equipment) because of failure of firefighting methods, late fire detection, undetected fires, or fire size.

During the first and fifth periods, the largest number of fires were suppressed with water alone. During the second period, the largest number of fires were suppressed manually with or without portable fire extinguishers. During the third period, the largest number of fires were suppressed with portable fire extinguishers or water alone and manually with or without portable fire extinguishers. During the fourth period, the largest number of fires were extinguished with portable fire extinguishers alone or together with dry chemical powder, foam, and water. During the sixth period, the largest number of fires were extinguished with portable fire extinguishers, dry chemical powder, foam, and water.

Equipment Involved

Table 42 shows the number of fires by equipment involved for each time period. The equipment most often involved was mobile equipment (dozers, loaders, trucks, tankers, drills, and shovels), oxyfuel torches (at times electrical arc welding equipment was used), heaters and burners, and maintenance equipment. Other equipment included facilities (considered equipment in this report), chemical/flammable liquid/gas tanks, beltlines, electrical control systems, a hopper, a crusher, a preheat system, a generator, a product treatment pot, and an explosive device. During the first, third, and fifth periods, the largest number of fires involved heaters, burners, and maintenance equipment. During the second period, the largest number of fires involved oxyfuel torches. During the fourth and

sixth periods, the largest number of fires involved mobile equipment.

Location

Table 43 shows the number of fires by location for each time period. The most common locations were flame cutting/welding areas, maintenance and refuse areas, and mobile equipment working areas (haulage, loading, mining, drilling, transportation, and crusher areas). Other fire locations included facility and garage areas, raw mills, preheat and storage silo areas, product treatment areas, beltline and hopper areas, and waste dump, pit, crusher, screen, and deck areas. Electrical control and power house areas, chemical and flammable liquid storage areas, and generator housing were also affected by the fires. During the first, third, and fifth periods, the largest number of fires occurred at maintenance and refuse areas. During the second period, the largest number of fires occurred at flame cutting/welding areas. During the fourth and sixth periods, the largest number of fires occurred at mobile equipment working areas.

Burning Materials

Table 44 shows the number of fires by burning material for each time period. The materials most often involved were oxyfuel/

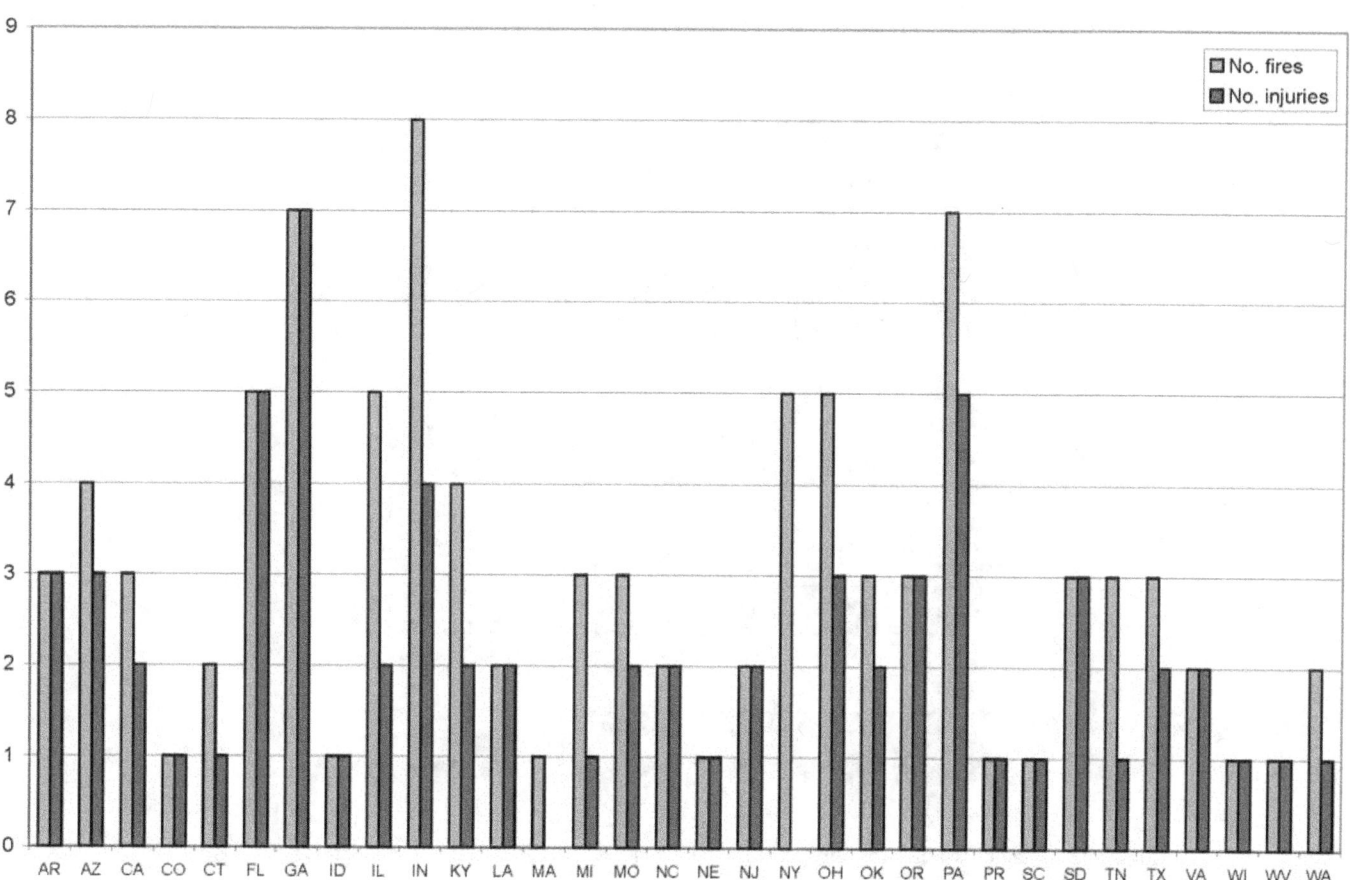

Figure 13.—Number of fires and fire injuries for surface stone mines by state, 1990–2001.

28

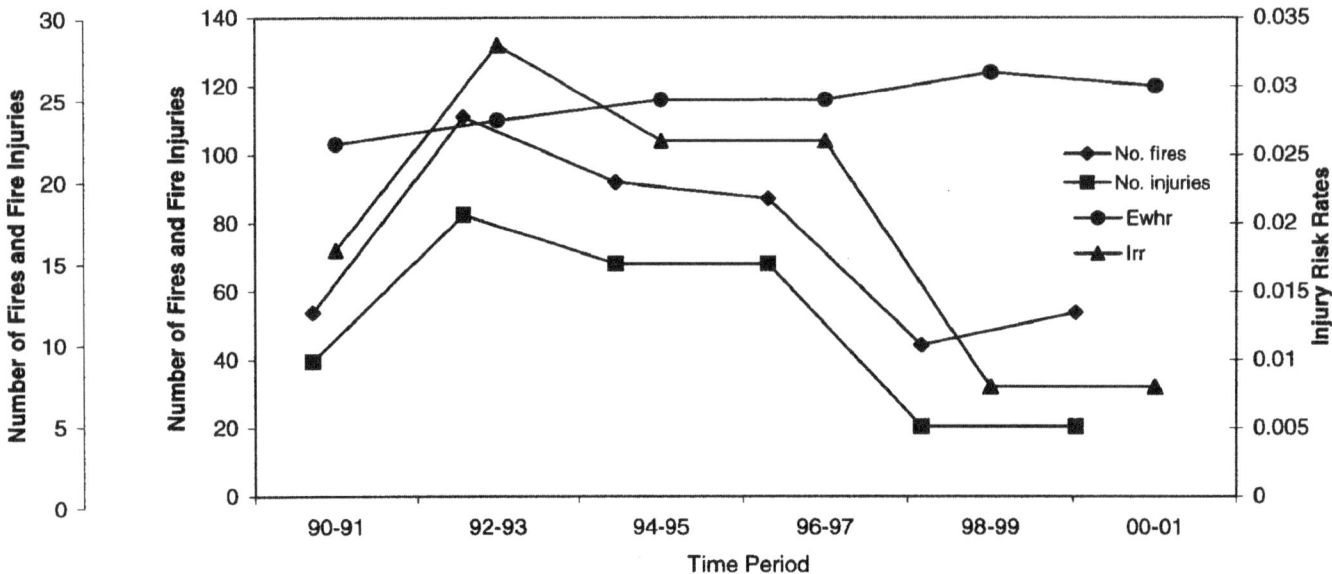

Figure 14.—Number of fires, fire injuries, risk rates, and employees' working hours for surface stone mines by time period, 1990–2001.

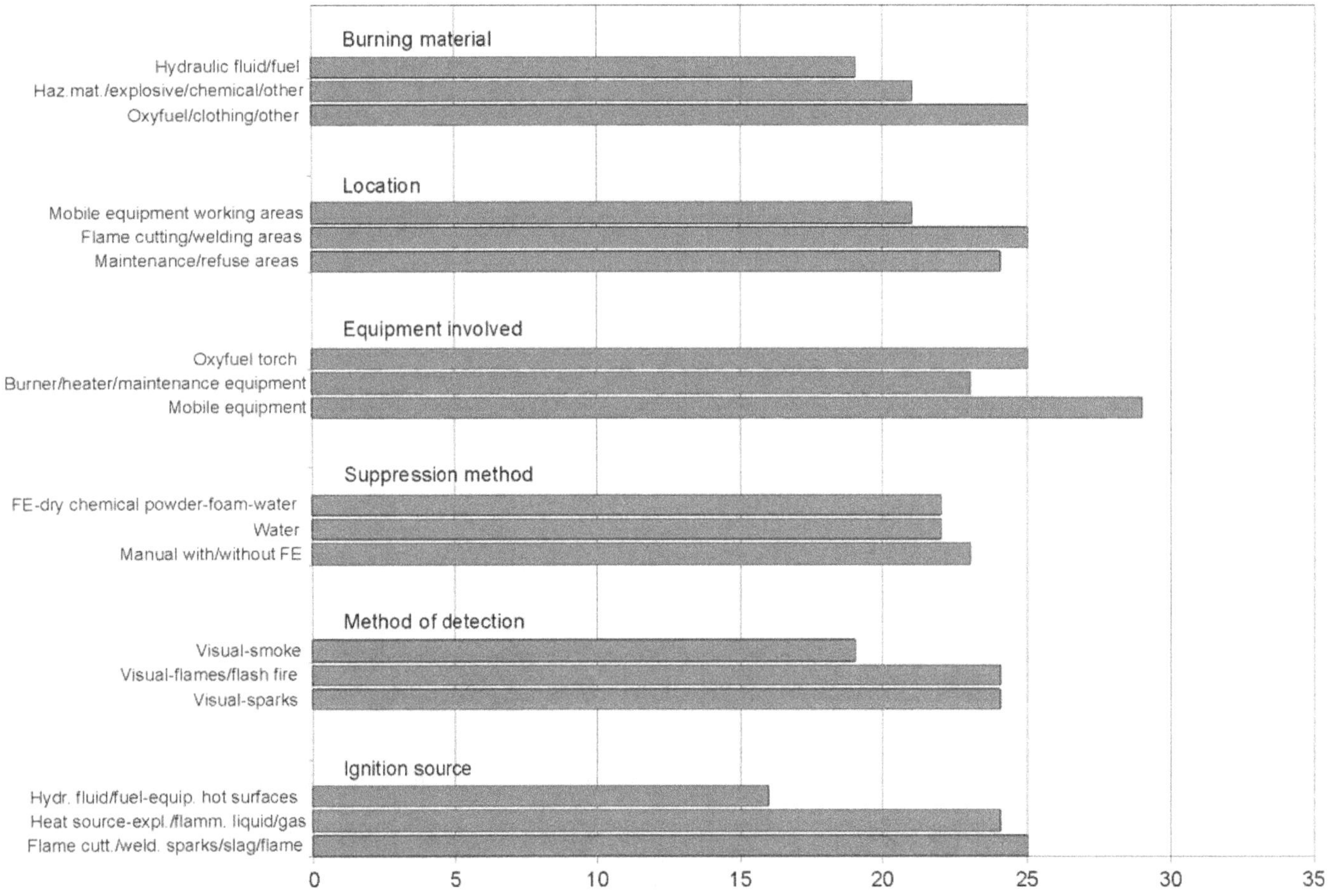

Figure 15.—Major variables for surface stone mine fires, 1990–2001. (FE = portable fire extinguisher)

Table 37.—Number of fires, fire injuries, and risk rates for surface stone mines by state,[1]
employees' working hours, and lost workdays, 1990–2001

State[2]	No. fires[2]	No. fire injuries[2]	LWD[3]	Ewhr,[3] 10^6 hr	Irr[4]
Arizona	4	3	26	5.8	0.014
Arkansas	3	3	52	14	0.043
California	3	2	20	21.6	0.019
Colorado	1	1	12	8.2	0.024
Connecticut	2	1	—	5.3	0.038
Florida	5	5	50	39.5	0.025
Georgia	7	7	115	24	0.058
Idaho	1	1	—	3.5	0.057
Illinois	5	2	247	24.6	0.016
Indiana	8	4	64	17.6	0.046
Kentucky	4	2	6	16.4	0.024
Louisiana	2	2	2	4.2	0.095
Massachusetts	1	—	—	8.2	—
Michigan	3	1	43	11.3	0.018
Missouri	3	2	18	28	0.014
Nebraska	1	1	—	2	0.1
New Jersey	2	2	150	10	0.04
New York	5	—	7	17	—
North Carolina	2	2	24	27	0.015
Ohio	5	3	49	22	0.027
Oklahoma	3	2	32	19.2	0.021
Oregon	3	3	38	14.7	0.041
Pennsylvania	7	5	177	46	0.022
Puerto Rico	1	1	30	11.4	0.018
South Carolina	1	1	24	7.5	0.027
South Dakota	3	3	15	5.4	0.111
Tennessee[5]	3	1	6,152	18	0.011
Texas	3	2	37	49	0.008
Virginia	2	2	—	21.7	0.018
Washington	2	1	—	5.2	0.039
West Virginia	1	1	—	6	0.033
Wisconsin	1	1	9	18	0.011
All other states	—	—	—	157	—
Total	97	67	7,399	689	[4]0.02

[1]Includes Puerto Rico.
[2]Derived from MSHA "Fire Accident Abstract" internal publications.
[3]Derived from MSHA "Injury Experience in Mining" publications.
[4]Calculated according to MSHA formula reported in the "Methodologies" section.
[5]Tennessee had 1 fire fatality caused by a hydraulic fluid/fuel fire involving a truck.

clothing/grease and other materials (including screen shaft, crusher, hopper, stampler breaker materials, rubber hoses, gear boxes, bin feeder, hydraulic fluid, and chute liner), hazardous materials, chemicals, oil, refuse, detonated explosives, and hydraulic fluid/fuel. Other burning materials included flammable liquids and gas, facilities and their contents, electrical wires and cables, belts and hot materials, equipment mechanical components, and deck liner.

During the first and fifth periods, the largest number of fires involved hazardous material, chemicals, refuse, oil, and detonated explosives. During the second period, the largest number of fires involved oxyfuel/clothing/grease and other materials. During the third period, the largest number of fires involved oxyfuel and hazardous materials. During the fourth and sixth periods, the largest number of fires involved hydraulic fluid/fuel.

Fire Injuries

Table 45 shows the number of fire injuries per number of fires causing injuries and total fires by year, ignition source, equipment involved, and location for 1990–2001. Overall, there were 67 injuries and 1 fatality caused by 68 fires. The greatest number of fire injuries occurred in 1993 (11 injuries and 1 fatality caused by 12 fires). The ignition sources that caused the greatest number of fire injuries were flame cutting/welding spark/slag/flame, heat source, and hydraulic fluid/fuel sprayed onto equipment hot surfaces. Other ignition sources were flammable liquid/refueling fuel on hot surfaces, electrical short/arcing, overheated oil, hot material, and mechanical friction. The equipment involved in fire injuries included oxyfuel torches, heaters, mobile equipment, maintenance equipment, electrical systems, air compressors, beltline, and kiln. The locations where most of the fire injuries occurred were flame cutting/welding areas, maintenance and refuse areas, and mobile equipment working areas. Other fire locations were generator housing, beltlines, and kiln areas.

A fatality occurred in Tennessee [MSHA 1993e], which was caused by a hydraulic fluid fire involving a truck. The victim was severely burned in the cab, probably due to the sudden ignition of flammable vapors and mists that penetrated the cab.

Table 38.—Number of fires, fire injuries, fire fatalities, and risk rates for surface stone mines
by time period, employees' working hours, and lost workdays, 1990–2001

	Time period						
	90-91	92-93	94-95	96-97	98-99	00-01	1990-2001
Number of fires[1]	12	24	20	19	10	12	97
Number of fire injuries[1]	9	18	15	15	5	5	67
Number of fire fatalities[1]	—	1	—	—	—	—	1
LWD[2]	191	6,133	784	155	57	79	7,399
Ewhr,[2] 10^6 hr	103	110	116	116	124	120	689
Irr[3]	0.018	0.033	0.026	0.026	0.008	0.008	[3]0.02

[1]Derived from MSHA "Fire Accident Abstract" internal publications.
[2]Derived from MSHA "Injury Experience in Mining" publications.
[3]Calculated according to MSHA formula reported in the "Methodologies" section.

Table 39.—Number of fires for surface stone mines by ignition source and time period, 1990–2001

	Time period						
Ignition source	90-91 No. fires	92-93 No. fires	94-95 No. fires	96-97 No. fires	98-99 No. fires	00-01 No. fires	1990-2001 No. fires
Flame cutting/welding spark/slag/flame	3	10	5	3	2	2	25
Heat source/explosion-flammable liquid/gas	5	4	6	4	4	1	24
Hydraulic fluid/fuel on equipment hot surfaces	2	4	2	3	—	5	16
Electrical short/arcing	—	—	2	4	—	1	7
Refueling fuel/flammable liquid on hot surfaces	—	1	2	—	2	—	5
Explosion/ignition-hazardous material/chemical/ explosives/flammable gas	—	1	1	1	1	—	4
Hot material	—	—	1	1	1	—	3
Overheated oil	—	1	—	1	—	—	2
Engine malfunction/mechanical friction	—	—	—	1	—	1	2
Unknown	2	3	1	1	—	2	9
Total	12	24	20	19	10	12	97

Table 40.—Number of fires for surface stone mines by method of detection and time period,
1990–2001

	Time period						
Method of detection	90-91 No. fires	92-93 No. fires	94-95 No. fires	96-97 No. fires	98-99 No. fires	00-01 No. fires	1990-2001 No. fires
Visual:							
Flames/flash fires	2	5	5	3	3	6	24
Sparks	3	10	5	3	2	1	24
Smoke	—	3	4	6	4	2	19
Late smoke detection	—	2	—	2	—	—	4
White mist	—	—	—	—	—	1	1
Heard an explosion	3	1	2	2	1	—	9
Touched a hot spot	2	1	3	2	—	—	8
Undetected	2	2	1	1	—	2	8
Total	12	24	20	19	10	12	97

Table 41.—Number of fires for surface stone mines by suppression method and time period,
1990–2001

	Time period						
Suppression method	90-91 No. fires	92-93 No. fires	94-95 No. fires	96-97 No. fires	98-99 No. fires	00-01 No. fires	1990-2001 No. fires
Manual with or without FE[1]	3	10	5	3	2	—	23
Water	4	4	5	4	4	1	22
FE-DCP-foam-water	2	5	4	5	2	4	22
FE	1	2	5	5	2	3	18
Destroyed/HD[2]	2	3	1	2	—	4	12
Total	12	24	20	19	10	12	97

DCP   Dry chemical powder.
FE   Portable fire extinguisher.
HD   Heavily damaged.
[1]Method used by welders to extinguish clothing and oxyfuel/grease fires.
[2]Usually due to failure of firefighting methods, late fire detection, undetected fires, or fire size.

Table 42.—Number of fires for surface stone mines by equipment involved and time period, 1990–2001

Equipment	Time period						1990-2001
	90-91 No. fires	92-93 No. fires	94-95 No. fires	96-97 No. fires	98-99 No. fires	00-01 No. fires	No. fires
Mobile equipment[1]	2	5	5	7	3	7	29
Oxyfuel torch[2]	3	10	5	3	2	2	25
Heater/maintenance equipment/burner	4	4	6	4	4	1	23
Facilities[3]	2	3	1	1	—	—	7
Chemical/flammable liquid/gas tanks	—	—	1	1	1	—	3
Hopper/crusher/preheat system	—	—	—	2	1	—	3
Generator/product treatment pot	1	—	—	1	—	—	2
Beltlines	—	1	—	—	1	1	2
Electrical control system	—	—	1	—	—	1	2
Explosive device	—	1	—	—	—	—	1
Other	—	—	1	—	—	—	1
Total	12	24	20	19	10	12	97

[1]Includes dozers, loaders, trucks, drills, shovels, and tankers.
[2]At times, electrical arc welding equipment was used.
[3]Considered equipment in this report.

Table 43.—Number of fires for surface stone mines by location and time period, 1990–2001

Location	Time period						1990-2001
	90-91 No. fires	92-93 No. fires	94-95 No. fires	96-97 No. fires	98-99 No. fires	00-01 No. fires	No. fires
Flame cutting/welding areas[1]	3	10	5	3	2	2	25
Maintenance/refuse areas	4	4	7	4	5	—	24
Mobile equipment working areas[2]	2	4	3	6	1	5	21
Facility/garage areas	2	3	1	—	—	3	9
Raw mill/preheat/silo/product treatment areas	1	—	2	1	1	—	5
Waste dump/pit/crusher/screen deck areas	—	2	—	1	—	1	4
Beltline/hopper areas	—	1	1	1	—	1	4
Chemical/flammable liquid storage areas	—	—	—	1	1	—	2
Electrical control/power house areas	—	—	1	1	—	—	2
Generator housing	—	—	—	1	—	—	1
Total	12	24	20	19	10	12	97

[1]Includes generator housing, chute, deck, bin feeder, crusher, hopper, shop, stampler breaker and screen shaft areas, and maintenance areas.
[2]Includes haulage, loading, mining, drilling, transportation, and crusher areas.

Table 44.—Number of fires for surface stone mines by burning material and time period, 1990–2001

Burning material	Time period						1990-2001
	90-91 No. fires	92-93 No. fires	94-95 No. fires	96-97 No. fires	98-99 No. fires	00-01 No. fires	No. fires
Oxyfuel/clothing/grease/other[1]	3	10	5	3	2	2	25
Hazardous material/chemical/refuse/oil/ detonated explosive	4	5	5	3	4	—	21
Hydraulic fluid/fuel/oil	2	4	2	6	—	5	19
Flammable liquid/gas	1	1	4	1	3	—	10
Facility/content	2	3	1	—	—	1	7
Electrical wires/cables	—	—	2	4	—	1	7
Belt/hot material	—	1	1	1	1	1	5
Equipment mechanical components	—	—	—	1	—	1	2
Deck liner	—	—	—	—	—	1	1
Total	12	24	20	19	10	12	97

[1]Includes screen shaft, crusher and hopper, stampler breaker, chute liner, hydraulic fluid, rubber hoses, gear boxes, and bin feeder.

Table 45.—Number of fire injuries per number of fires causing injuries and total fires for surface stone mines by year, ignition source, equipment involved, and location, 1990–2001

Year	No. total fires	No. fires causing injuries	No. fire injuries	Ignition source	Equipment	Location
1990 . . .	6	4	2	Heat source	Heater	Refuse pile area.
			2	Flame cutting/welding spark/slag/flame	Oxyfuel torch	Flame cutting/welding areas.[1]
1991 . . .	6	5	2	Heat source	Heater	Maintenance area.
			1	Flame cutting/welding spark/slag/flame	Oxyfuel torch	Flame cutting/welding areas.[1]
			1	Flammable gas explosion	Product treatment pot	Product treatment areas.
			1	Hydraulic fluid/fuel on equipment hot surfaces	Loader	Loading area.
1992 . . .	10	7	5	Flame cutting/welding spark/slag/flame	Oxyfuel torch	Flame cutting/welding areas.[1]
			1	Heat source	Heater	Maintenance area.
			1	Overheated oil	Air compressor	Drilling area.
1993[2] . .	14	12	5	Flame cutting/welding spark/slag/flame	Oxyfuel torch	Flame cutting/welding areas.[1]
			3	Heat source	Heater	Beltline/refuse pile areas.
			2	Hydraulic fluid/fuel on equipment hot surfaces	Truck/dozer	Crusher/mining areas.
			1	Refueling fuel on hot surfaces	Truck	Maintenance area.
1994 . . .	9	6	3	Flame cutting/welding spark/slag/flame	Oxyfuel torch	Flame cutting/welding areas.[1]
			2	Heat source	Heater	Maintenance area.
			1	Hydraulic fluid/fuel on equipment hot surfaces	Loader	Loading area.
1995 . . .	11	9	4	Heat source	Heater	Hopper belt/maintenance areas.
			2	Flame cutting/welding spark/slag/flame	Oxyfuel torch	Flame cutting/welding areas.[1]
			2	Flammable liquid on hot surfaces	Truck/loader	Maintenance area.
			1	Electrical short/arcing	Dozer cab	Mining area.
1996 . . .	12	9	2	Heat source	Heater	Maintenance area.
			2	Electrical short/arcing	Generator/truck	Generator housing/haulage area.
			1	Flame cutting/welding spark/slag	Oxyfuel torch	Flame cutting/welding areas.[1]
			3	Hydraulic fluid/fuel on equipment hot surfaces	Dozer/truck	Mining/haulage areas.
			1	Oil on hot surfaces	Truck	—
1997 . . .	7	6	1	Mechanical friction	Loader	Loading area.
			2	Flame cutting/welding spark/slag/flame	Oxyfuel torch	Flame cutting/welding areas.[1]
			2	Heat source	Heater	Maintenance/working areas.
			1	Hot material	Hopper belt	Hopper area.
1998 . . .	4	4	1	Heat source	Heater	Maintenance area.
			1	Flammable liquid on hot surfaces	Truck	Preheat tower.
			1	Hot material	Kiln	Kiln area.
			1	Flame cutting/welding spark/slag/flame	Oxyfuel torch	Flame cutting/welding areas.[1]
1999 . . .	6	1	1	Fuel on hot surfaces	—	Storage shed.
2000 . . .	4	3	1	Hydraulic fluid/fuel on equipment hot surfaces	Truck	Haulage area.
			1	Flame cutting/welding spark/slag/flame	Shovel	Flame cutting/welding areas.[1]
			1	Electrical short/arcing	Loader	Loading area.
2001 . . .	8	2	1	Flame cutting/welding spark/slag/flame	Oxyfuel/torch	Flame cutting/welding areas.[1]
			1	Heat source	Gas heater	Screen deck.
Total . . .	97	68	67			

[1]Includes crusher, ball chain, bin feeder, screen shaft, stamper breaker and beltline areas, and mobile equipment maintenance areas.
[2]In 1993, there was 1 fire fatality, which was caused by a hydraulic fluid/fuel fire involving a truck.

METAL/NONMETAL MILL FIRES

Table 46 and figure 16 show the number of fires and fire injuries for metal/nonmetal mills by state during 1990–2001. Table 46 also shows the injury risk rates, employees' working hours, and lost workdays. In all, 77 fires occurred in 26 states. Thirty-seven of the fires caused 41 injuries and 1 fatality (including 5 fires and 3 injuries involving contractors). The yearly average was 6.4 fires and 3.4 injuries. Fifty-four fires with 26 injuries and 1 fatality occurred at metal mills; 23 fires with 15 injuries occurred at nonmetal mills. The Ewhr value was 845×10^6 hr (Irr = 0.01), and the LWD value was 6,681.

Minnesota had the most fires (16 fires and 5 injuries), followed by Arizona (9 fires and 3 injuries), Wyoming (8 fires and 3 injuries), Nevada (7 fires, 4 injuries, and 1 fatality), and Texas (4 fires and 7 injuries). Of these states, Texas had the highest injury risk rate value (Irr = 0.033).

Table 47, partly illustrated in figure 17, shows the number of fires, fire injuries, fire fatalities, risk rates, employees' working hours, and lost workdays by time period. The number of fires increased slightly during the second period, then decreased during the remaining periods. The number of fire injuries show a decrease during most of the periods (an increase is seen during the third period), accompanied by a decline in employees' working hours during most of the periods. The Irr values follow patterns similar to those shown by the injury values.

Tables 48–53 show the number of fires by ignition source, method of detection and suppression, equipment involved, location, and burning material by time period. Figure 18 shows the major variables related to fires for 1990–2001. Table 54 shows the number of fire injuries per number of fires causing injuries and total fires by year, ignition source, equipment involved, and location.

Ignition Source

Table 48 shows the number of fires and injuries by ignition source for each time period. The leading sources were flame cutting/welding spark/slag/flame (29 fires or 38%), hot material (12 fires or 16%), and flammable liquid/oil/refueling fuel on hot surfaces/explosion (9 fires or 11%). Other ignition sources were electrical short/arcing, conveyor belt friction, overheated oil, surface vaporized oil on hot surface, chemical explosion/ignition, hydraulic fluid/fuel sprayed onto equipment hot surfaces, and heat source. Two sources were unknown. At least one of the three mobile equipment hydraulic fluid/fuel fires became a large fire because of continuous flow of fluids from the pump due to engine shutoff failure. In this instance, the cab was suddenly engulfed in flames, probably due to the ignition of flammable vapors and mists that penetrated the cab.

During the first, third, fourth, and fifth periods, the largest number of fires were caused by flame cutting/welding spark/slag/flame. During the second period, the largest number of fires were caused by flammable liquid/oil/refueling fuel on hot surfaces/explosion. During the sixth period, the largest number of fires were caused by flame cutting/welding spark/slag/flame, conveyor belt friction, and overheated oil.

Method of Detection

Table 49 shows the number of fires by method of detection for each time period. The most frequent methods were workers who saw smoke long after the fires had started, followed by welders who saw sparks and operators who saw the fires when they started as flames/flash fires. Other methods of detection were workers who saw smoke shortly after the fires had started, workers who heard an electric trip warning or an explosion, workers who saw a smoldering fire, and an operator who saw white smoke. Four fires were undetected.

During the first period, the largest number of fires were detected by workers as smoke long after the fires had started, by operators as flames/flash fires, and by welders as sparks. During the second, fourth, and fifth periods, the largest number of fires were detected by workers as smoke long after the fires had started. During the third period, the largest number of fires were detected by operators as flames/flash fires. During the sixth period, the largest number of fires were detected by workers as smoke.

Suppression Method

Table 50 shows the number of fires by suppression method for each time period. The most common methods were water or portable fire extinguishers alone and manual techniques with or without portable fire extinguishers. None of the equipment involved in fires had machine fire suppression systems. Other suppression methods were portable fire extinguishers with foam, dry chemical powder, and water. On at least five occasions, including one mobile equipment fire, fire brigades and fire departments fought the fires with portable fire extinguishers together with foam, dry chemical, and water. However, six fires

destroyed or heavily damaged equipment (including one piece of mobile equipment) because of failure of firefighting methods, late fire detection, undetected fires, or fire size.

During the first period, the largest number of fires were suppressed with water or portable fire extinguishers alone and manually with or without portable fire extinguishers. During the second period, the largest number of fires were suppressed with portable fire extinguishers alone. During the third through fifth periods, the largest number of fires were extinguished with water alone. During the sixth period, the largest number of fires were extinguished with water or portable fire extinguishers.

Equipment Involved

Table 51 shows the number of fires by equipment involved for each time period. The equipment most often involved was oxyfuel torches (at times electrical arc welding equipment was used). This was followed by dust collectors, air compressors, chutes, dryers, crushers, liquor and refueling pumps, and oil vaporizers. Other equipment included mobile equipment (trucks, dozers, loaders, shovels, and forklifts), beltlines, and electrical breakers, cathodes, and fixtures. Also involved in fires were facilities (considered equipment in this report), heaters, sample and chemical containers, a hydroprecipitator, kilns, product cooling systems, and maintenance equipment.

During the first, third, fourth, and fifth periods, the largest number of fires involved oxyfuel torches. During the second period, the largest number of fires involved oxyfuel torches, mobile equipment, dust collectors, air compressors, chutes, crushers, and dryers. During the sixth period, the largest number of fires involved oxyfuel torches and dust collectors.

Location

Table 52 shows the number of fires by location for each time period. The most common locations were flame cutting/welding areas, beltline areas, and maintenance areas. Other fire locations included dust collectors, air compressors, chutes, crushers, dryers, pelletizer building, baghouse, refinery, liquor pump areas, storage silos, product cooling areas, boiler rooms, power houses, and chemical storage areas. Mobile equipment working areas (haulage, loading, and mining areas), facility and elevator shaft, and a lab and shop were also affected by the fires. During the first through fifth periods, the largest number of fires occurred at flame cutting/welding areas. During the sixth period, the largest number of fires occurred at flame cutting/welding areas, dust collectors, and maintenance areas.

Burning Materials

Table 53 shows the number of fires by burning material for each time period. The materials most often involved were oxyfuel/clothing/grease and other materials (including liquor pumps, belt material, pipelines, dust collector and chute liners, flammable liquids, wood pallets, crusher and screen panel). This was followed by belt and hot materials, flammable liquids, refueling fuel, and vaporized oil. Other burning materials included electrical wires and cables, facilities and their contents, and oil, chemicals, refuse, and core samples. Dust collector and chute liners, pipeline and crusher materials, equipment mechanical components, and hydraulic fluid/fuel were also involved in the fires.

During the first, third, fourth, and fifth periods, the largest number of fires involved oxyfuel/clothing/grease and other materials. During the second period, the largest number of fires involved oxyfuel and flammable liquids, refueling fuel, and vaporized oil. During the sixth period, the largest number of fires involved oxyfuel, flammable liquids, and facilities and their content.

Fire Injuries

Table 54 shows the number of fire injuries per number of fires causing injuries and total fires by year, ignition source, equipment involved, and location for 1990–2001. Overall, there were 41 injuries and 1 fatality caused by 37 fires.

The greatest number of fire injuries occurred in 1990 (eight injuries caused by eight fires) and 1994 (seven injuries and one fatality caused by six fires). The ignition sources that caused the injuries were flame cutting/welding spark/slag/flame, flammable liquid/refueling fuel on hot surfaces/explosion, and hot material. Other ignition sources were chemical ignition, electrical short/arcing, overheated oil, conveyor belt friction, heat source, and hydraulic fluid/fuel sprayed onto equipment hot surfaces. The equipment involved in fire injuries included oxyfuel torches, maintenance equipment, refueling and liquor pumps, and product cooling systems. Other equipment included chemical containers, electrical systems, air compressors, mobile equipment, heaters, and beltline. The location where most of the fire injuries occurred were the flame cutting/welding areas, maintenance areas, pump housing, liquor pump and refinery areas, and product cooling area. Other fire locations were lab and storage areas, crusher and pelletizer building, beltline, maintenance areas, and mobile equipment working areas.

A fatality occurred in Nevada [MSHA 1994e]. The victim, equipped with firefighting gear and self-contained breathing apparatus, was fighting a refinery electrical fire. The victim was found unconscious on the floor.

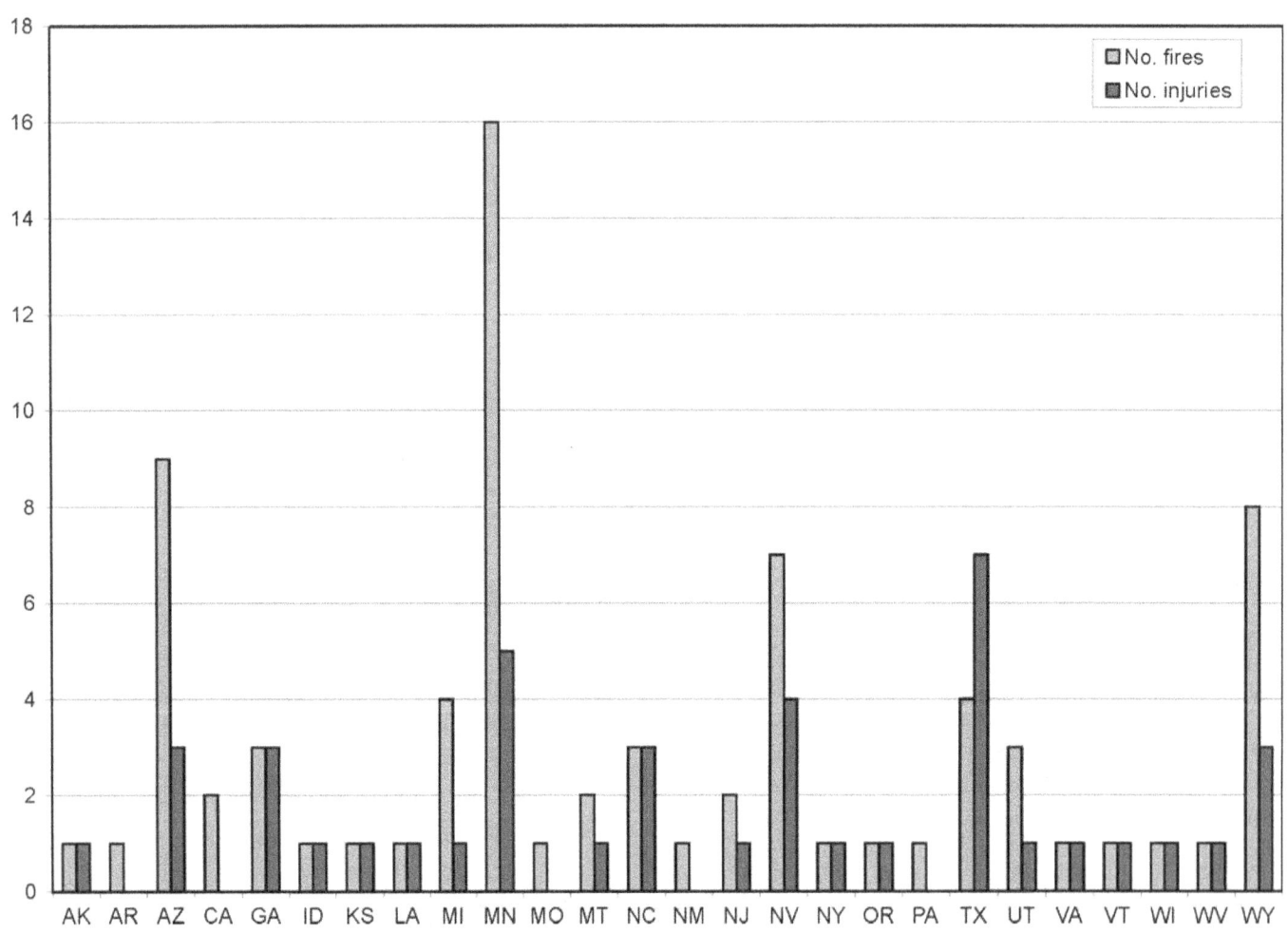

Figure 16.—Number of fires and fire injuries for metal/nonmetal mills by state, 1990–2001.

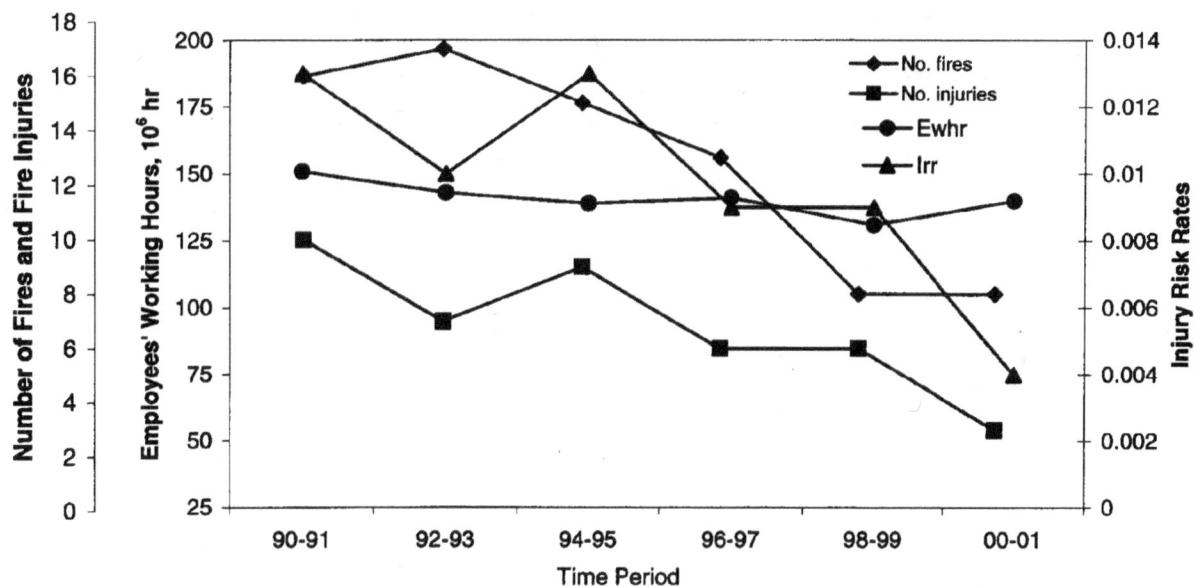

Figure 17.—Number of fires, fire injuries, risk rates, and employees' working hours for metal/nonmetal mills by time period, 1990–2001.

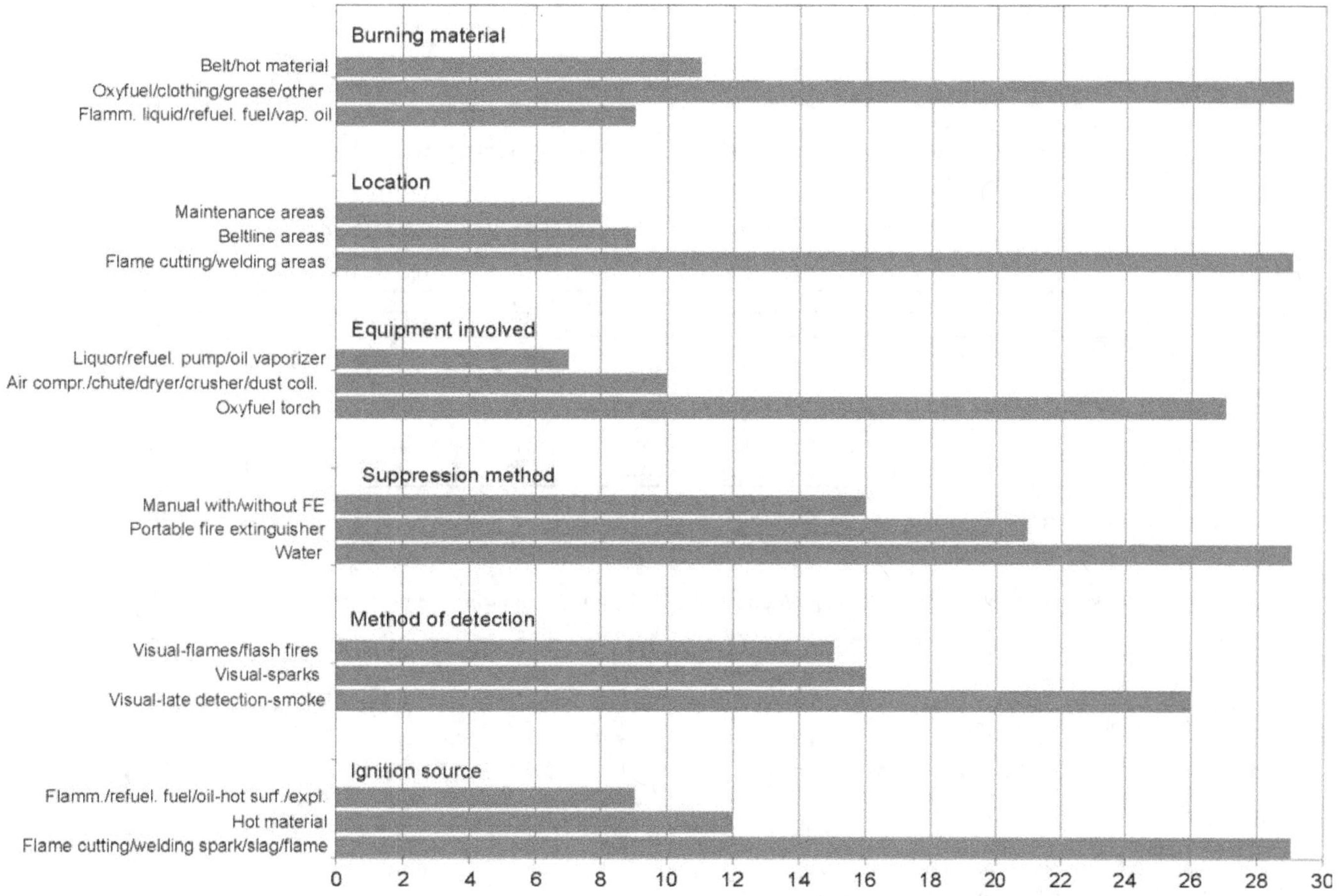

Figure 18.—Major variables for metal/nonmetal mill fires, 1990–2001. (FE = portable fire extinguisher)

Table 46.—Number of fires, fire injuries, and risk rates for metal/nonmetal mills by state, employees' working hours, and lost workdays, 1990–2001

State[1]	No. fires[1]	No. fire injuries[1]	LWD[2]	Ewhr,[2] 10^6 hr	Irr[3]
Alaska	1	1	7	7.1	0.028
Arizona	9	3	56	78.5	0.008
Arkansas	1	—	—	18.5	—
California	2	—	—	44.72	—
Georgia	3	3	6	102	0.006
Idaho	1	1	—	7	0.029
Kansas	1	1	33	4.5	0.044
Louisiana	1	1	50	16.5	0.012
Michigan	4	1	11	27	0.007
Minnesota	16	5	26	75	0.013
Missouri	1	—	—	4.8	—
Montana	2	1	—	33.5	0.006
Nevada[4]	7	4	6,058	86	0.009
New Jersey	2	1	—	0.65	0.308
New Mexico	1	—	—	11.4	—
New York	1	1	18	1.2	0.17
North Carolina	3	3	—	16.4	0.037
Oregon	1	1	—	1.84	0.109
Pennsylvania	1	—	—	2	—
Texas	4	7	385	42	0.033
Utah	3	1	—	26.4	0.008
Vermont	1	1	9	1.63	0.123
Virginia	1	1	—	7.9	0.025
West Virginia	1	1	—	0.6	0.333
Wisconsin	1	—	—	0.2	—
Wyoming	8	3	22	46.1	0.013
All other states	—	—	—	182	—
Total	77	41	6,681	845	[3]0.01

[1]Derived from MSHA "Fire Accident Abstract" internal publications.
[2]Derived from MSHA "Injury Experience in Mining" publications.
[3]Calculated according to MSHA formula reported in the "Methodologies" section.
[4]Nevada had 1 fire fatality.

Table 47.—Number of fires, fire injuries, fire fatalities, and risk rates for metal/nonmetal mills by time period, employees' working hours, and lost workdays, 1990–2001

	Time period						
	90-91	92-93	94-95	96-97	98-99	00-01	1990-2001
Number of fires[1]	16	17	15	13	8	8	77
Number of fire injuries[1]	10	7	9	6	6	3	41
Number of fire fatalities[1]	—	—	1	—	—	—	1
LWD[2]	58	78	6,033	50	411	51	6,681
Ewhr,[2] 10^6 hr	151	143	139	141	131	140	845
Irr[3]	0.013	0.010	0.013	0.009	0.009	0.004	[3]0.01

[1]Derived from MSHA "Fire Accident Abstract" internal publications.
[2]Derived from MSHA "Injury Experience in Mining" publications.
[3]Calculated according to MSHA formula reported in the "Methodologies" section.

Table 48.—Number of fires for metal/nonmetal mills by ignition source and time period, 1990–2001

Ignition source	Time period						
	90-91 No. fires	92-93 No. fires	94-95 No. fires	96-97 No. fires	98-99 No. fires	00-01 No. fires	1990-2001 No. fires
Flame cutting/welding spark/slag/flame	7	4	8	5	3	2	29
Hot material	1	3	3	3	2	—	12
Flammable liquid/refueling fuel/oil on hot surfaces/ explosion	3	5	—	—	—	1	9
Electrical short/arcing	3	1	1	1	2	—	8
Conveyor belt friction	1	2	—	2	—	2	7
Overheated/vaporized oil on hot surface	1	1	—	—	—	2	4
Hydraulic fluid/fuel on equipment hot surfaces	—	1	—	1	—	—	2
Chemical explosion/ignition	—	—	1	—	1	—	2
Heat source	—	—	1	—	—	1	2
Unknown	—	—	1	1	—	—	2
Total	16	17	15	13	8	8	77

Table 49.—Number of fires for metal/nonmetal mills by method of detection and time period, 1990–2001

Method of detection	Time period						1990-2001
	90-91 No. fires	92-93 No. fires	94-95 No. fires	96-97 No. fires	98-99 No. fires	00-01 No. fires	No. fires
Visual:							
Late smoke detection	5	7	3	5	3	3	26
Sparks	5	3	3	2	2	1	16
Flames/flash fires	5	3	4	2	1	—	15
Smoke	—	1	1	2	1	4	9
White smoke	1	—	—	—	—	—	1
Smoldering fire	—	—	—	1	—	—	1
Heard an electrical trip warning	—	2	2	—	—	—	4
Heard an explosion	—	1	—	—	—	—	1
Undetected	—	—	2	1	1	—	4
Total	16	17	15	13	8	8	77

Table 50.—Number of fires for metal/nonmetal mills by suppression method and time period, 1990–2001

Suppression method	Time period						1990-2001
	90-91 No. fires	92-93 No. fires	94-95 No. fires	96-97 No. fires	98-99 No. fires	00-01 No. fires	No. fires
Water	5	5	6	7	3	3	29
FE	5	8	2	1	2	3	21
Manual with or without FE[1]	5	2	3	3	2	1	16
FE-DCP-foam-water	—	2	2	1	—	—	5
Destroyed/HD[2]	1	—	2	1	1	1	6
Total	16	17	15	13	8	8	77

DCP   Dry chemical powder.
FE   Portable fire extinguisher.
HD   Heavily damaged.
[1]Method used by welders to extinguish clothing and oxyfuel/grease fires.
[2]Usually due to failure of firefighting methods, late fire detection, undetected fires, or fire size.

Table 51.—Number of fires for metal/nonmetal mills by equipment involved and time period, 1990–2001

Equipment	Time period						1990-2001
	90-91 No. fires	92-93 No. fires	94-95 No. fires	96-97 No. fires	98-99 No. fires	00-01 No. fires	No. fires
Oxyfuel torch[1]	6	4	7	5	3	2	27
Dust collector/air compressor/chute/dryer/crusher	2	4	1	1	—	2	10
Liquor/refueling pump/oil vaporizer	2	3	1	—	1	—	7
Electrical cathode/breaker/fixture	2	—	1	1	2	—	6
Beltline	1	1	—	2	1	1	6
Mobile equipment[2]	—	4	—	1	—	1	6
Facility[3]	—	—	2	2	1	—	5
Heater	—	1	1	—	—	1	3
Sample/chemical containers/hydroprecipitator	1	—	2	—	—	—	3
Maintenance equipment	2	—	—	—	—	—	2
Kiln/product cooling system	—	—	—	1	—	1	2
Total	16	17	15	13	8	8	77

[1]At times, electrical arc welding equipment was used.
[2]Includes shovels, forklifts, dozers, loaders, and trucks.
[3]Considered equipment in this report.

Table 52.—Number of fires for metal/nonmetal mills by location and time period, 1990–2001

Location	Time period						
	90-91 No. fires	92-93 No. fires	94-95 No. fires	96-97 No. fires	98-99 No. fires	00-01 No. fires	1990-2001 No. fires
Flame cutting/welding areas[1]	7	4	8	5	3	2	29
Beltline areas	1	3	—	3	1	1	9
Dust collector/air compressor/chute/crusher/dryer areas	2	3	1	—	—	2	8
Maintenance areas	3	3	—	—	—	2	8
Pelletizer/baghouse/refinery/liquor pump areas	2	2	1	1	—	—	6
Storage silos	—	—	2	2	—	—	4
Product cooling area/boiler room/power house/chemical storage	—	—	1	—	2	1	4
Mobile equipment working areas[2]	—	2	—	1	—	—	3
Facility/elevator shaft	—	—	1	1	1	—	3
Laboratory/shop	—	—	1	—	1	—	2
Other	1	—	—	—	—	—	1
Total	16	17	15	13	8	8	77

[1]Includes dust collector, chute and hopper areas, bin feeder, baghouse, pelletizer building, pipeline, elevator shaft, liquor pump, shops, beltline area, and maintenance areas.
[2]Includes haulage, loading, and mining areas.

Table 53.—Number of fires for metal/nonmetal mills by burning material and time period, 1990–2001

Burning material	Time period						
	90-91 No. fires	92-93 No. fires	94-95 No. fires	96-97 No. fires	98-99 No. fires	00-01 No. fires	1990-2001 No. fires
Oxyfuel/clothing/grease/other[1]	7	4	8	5	3	2	29
Belt/hot material	1	3	1	3	2	1	11
Flammable liquid/refueling fuel/vaporized oil	3	4	—	—	—	2	9
Electrical wires/cables	3	1	1	1	2	—	8
Oil/chemicals/refuse/core samples	1	1	2	1	—	—	5
Facility/content	—	—	2	1	1	2	6
Dust collector/chute liners/pipeline/crusher material	1	1	1	1	—	—	4
Hydraulic fluid/fuel	—	1	—	1	—	—	2
Equipment mechanical components	—	2	—	—	—	1	3
Total	16	17	15	13	8	8	77

[1]Includes liquor pumps, belt material, pipelines, flammable liquids, dust collector and chute liners, wood pallets, crusher, and screen panel.

Table 54.—Number of fire injuries per number of fires causing injuries and total fires for metal/nonmetal mills by year, ignition source, equipment involved, and location, 1990–2001

Year	No. total fires	No. fires causing injuries	No. fire injuries	Ignition source	Equipment	Location
1990	12	8	4	Flame cutting/welding spark/slag/flame	Oxyfuel torch	Flame cutting/welding areas.
			2	Electrical short/arcing	Electrical system	Crusher/pelletizer building.
			2	Flammable liquid on hot surfaces	Maintenance equipment	Maintenance area.
1991	4	2	1	Flame cutting/welding spark/slag/flame	Oxyfuel torch	Flame cutting/welding areas.
			1	Refueling fuel on hot surfaces	Refueling pump	Pump housing.
1992	8	2	1	Flame cutting/welding spark/slag/flame	Oxyfuel torch	Flame cutting/welding areas.
			1	Overheated oil	Air compressor	Mining area.
1993	9	5	2	Flame cutting/welding spark/slag/flame	Oxyfuel torch	Flame cutting/welding areas.
			3	Flammable liquid/refueling fuel on hot surfaces/explosion.	Liquor pump/heater/forklift	Maintenance area/liquor pump area.
1994[1]	10	6	3	Chemical ignition	Chemical samples	Storage/laboratory.
			1	Electrical short/arcing	Electrical system	Refinery building.
			3	Flame cutting/welding spark/slag/flame	Oxyfuel torch	Flame cutting/welding areas.
1995	5	2	2	Flame cutting/welding spark/slag/flame	Oxyfuel torch	Flame cutting/welding areas.
1996	8	3	1	Flame cutting/welding spark/slag/flame	Oxyfuel torch	Flame cutting/welding areas.
			1	Conveyor belt friction	Beltline	Beltline areas.
			1	Hydraulic fluid/fuel on equipment hot surfaces	Loader	Loading area.
1997	5	3	3	Flame cutting/welding spark/slag/flame	Oxyfuel torch	Flame cutting/welding areas.
1998	5	1	1	Chemical ignition	Chemical samples container	Laboratory.
1999	3	2	1	Flame cutting/welding spark/slag/flame	Oxyfuel torch	Flame cutting/welding areas.
			4	Hot material	Cooling system	Product cooling area.
2000	4	1	1	Flame cutting/welding spark/slag/flame	Oxyfuel torch	Flame cutting/welding areas.
2001	4	2	1	Oil on hot surfaces	Oil cooler	Power house.
			1	Heat source	Heater	Working area.
Total	77	37	41			

[1]In 1994, there was 1 fire fatality, which was caused by a refinery electrical fire.

STONE MILL FIRES

Table 55 and figure 19 show the number of fires and fire injuries for stone mills by state during 1990–2001. Table 55 also shows the injury risk rates, employees' working hours, and lost workdays. In all, 118 fires occurred in 33 states. Seventy-six of the fires caused 82 injuries (including 8 fires and 6 injuries involving contractors). The yearly average was 9.8 fires and 6.8 injuries. The Ewhr value was 873×10^6 hr (Irr = 0.019), and the LWD value was 1,911. Missouri had the most fires (16 fires and 9 injuries), followed by Pennsylvania (15 fires and 14 injuries), Michigan (9 fires and 5 injuries), and Virginia (7 fires and 5 injuries). Of these states, Virginia had the highest injury risk rate value (Irr = 0.091).

Table 56, partly illustrated in figure 20, shows the number of fires, fire injuries, risk rates, employees' working hours, and lost workdays by time period. The number of fires and fire injuries decreased during most of the periods, with a sharp increase during the last period. The number of employees' working hours increased throughout the periods. The Irr values follow patterns similar to those shown by the injury values.

Tables 57–63 show the number of fires by ignition source, method of detection and suppression, equipment involved, location, and burning material by time period. Figure 21 shows the major variables related to fires for 1990–2001. Table 63 shows the fire injuries per number of fires causing injuries and total fires by year, ignition source, equipment involved, and location.

Ignition Source

Table 57 shows the number of fires and fire injuries by ignition source for each time period. The leading sources were flame cutting/welding spark/slag/flame (53 fires or 45%), hot material (24 fires or 20%), and electrical short/arcing (11 fires or 9%). Other ignition sources were refueling fuel/flammable liquid/gas on hot surfaces/collision, heat source, hydraulic fluid/fuel sprayed onto equipment hot surfaces, conveyor belt friction, and overheated oil. One ignition source was unknown. At least four of the five mobile equipment hydraulic fluid/fuel fires became large fires because of the continuous flow of fluids from the pumps due to engine shutoff failure, difficulty in activating available emergency systems at ground level, lack of an emergency line drainage system, or lack of effective and rapid local firefighting response capabilities. In at least one instance, the cab was suddenly engulfed in flames, probably due to the ignition of flammable vapors and mists that penetrated the cab. Of note is that the hydraulic fluid fires subsequently involved the fuel system.

During the first, second, and fourth periods, the largest number of fires were caused by flame cutting/welding spark/slag/flame. During the third and sixth periods, the largest number of fires were caused by hot material. During the fifth period, the largest number of fires were caused by hot material and electrical short/arcing.

Method of Detection

Table 58 shows the number of fires by method of detection for each time period. The most frequent methods were welders who saw sparks, workers who saw smoke shortly and long after the fires had started, and operators who saw the fires when they started as flames/flash fires. Other methods of detection were workers who heard an explosion and workers who saw a glow or a smoldering fire. Six fires were undetected. The hot material fires were detected long after they had started due to lack of combustion smoke/gas detection systems.

During the first, second, and fourth periods, the largest number of fires were detected by welders as sparks. During the third and fifth periods, the largest number of fires were detected by workers as smoke long after the fires had started. During the sixth period, the largest number of fires were detected by operators as flames/flash fires.

Suppression Method

Table 59 shows the number of fires by suppression method for each time period. The most common methods were manual techniques with or without portable fire extinguishers, followed by water or portable fire extinguishers alone. Other suppression methods were portable fire extinguishers with foam, dry chemical powder, and water. One piece of mobile equipment involved in a fire had a machine fire suppression system, whose activation together with the engine shutoff system succeeded in temporarily abating the fire.

In at least 11 instances, including 2 mobiles equipment fires, fire brigades and fire departments fought the fires with portable fire extinguishers together with foam, dry chemical powder, and water. However, seven fires destroyed or heavily damaged equipment (including one piece of mobile equipment) because of failure of firefighting methods, late fire detection, undetected fires, or fire size.

During the first, second, and fourth periods, the largest number of fires were suppressed manually with or without portable fire extinguishers. During the third period, the largest number of fires were suppressed manually with or without portable fire extinguishers or water alone. During the fifth period, the largest number of fires were extinguished with water alone. During the sixth period, the largest number of fires were extinguished with water alone and portable fire extinguishers with foam, dry chemical powder, and water.

Equipment Involved

Table 60 shows the number of fires by equipment involved for each time period. The equipment most often involved were oxyfuel torches (at times electrical arc welding equipment was used), followed by kilns, preheat and cooling systems, and mobile equipment (loaders, trucks, drills, and locomotives). Other equipment included electrical systems, heaters, barrels, refueling pumps, beltlines, chutes, crushers, waste fuel tanks, dust collectors, and storage bins. Maintenance equipment and facilities (considered equipment in this report) were also involved in the fires.

During the first through fourth periods, the largest number of fires involved oxyfuel torches. During the fifth period, the largest number of fires involved electrical systems. During the sixth period, the largest number of fires involved oxyfuel torches, kilns, and preheat and cooling systems.

Location

Table 61 shows the number of fires by location for each time period. The most common locations were flame cutting/welding areas (at hopper, crusher, elevator shaft, chute and kiln areas, and maintenance areas). This was followed by kilns, hoppers, chutes, storage silo areas, mobile equipment working areas (shop and crusher areas, drilling, loading, haulage, transportation, and fuel preparation room), and beltline areas. Other fire locations included maintenance areas, pump and bagging stations, preheat and cooling areas, pit and bin areas, waste fuel areas, electrical control rooms, shops, and substation areas. Dust collector, crusher, chute, and facility areas were also affected by the fires.

During the first, second, and fourth periods, the largest number of fires occurred at flame cutting/welding areas. During the third period, the largest number of fires occurred at flame cutting/welding areas, kilns, chutes, hoppers, and storage silo areas. During the fifth period, the largest number of fires

occurred at beltline areas. During the sixth period, the largest number of fires occurred at kiln areas.

Burning Materials

Table 62 shows the number of fires by burning material for each time period. The materials most often involved were oxyfuels/ clothing/grease and other materials (including rubber hoses, pipelines, dust collector and chute liners, and shaft and kiln materials). This was followed by belt and kiln/clinker hot materials, flammable liquids/oil/refueling fuel, electrical wires/ cables/ transformers/ batteries, and rubber tires/refuse/waste fuel. Other materials involved in fires were hydraulic fluid/fuel, chute and dust collector liners and hoppers, and facilities and their content.

During the first, second, and fourth periods, the largest number of fires involved oxyfuel/clothing/grease and other materials. During the third period, the largest number of fires involved oxyfuel and belt and kiln/clinker hot materials. During the sixth period, the largest number of fires involved oxyfuel and flammable liquids, oil, and refueling fuel.

Fire Injuries

Table 63 shows the number of fire injuries per number of fires causing injuries and total fires by year, ignition source,

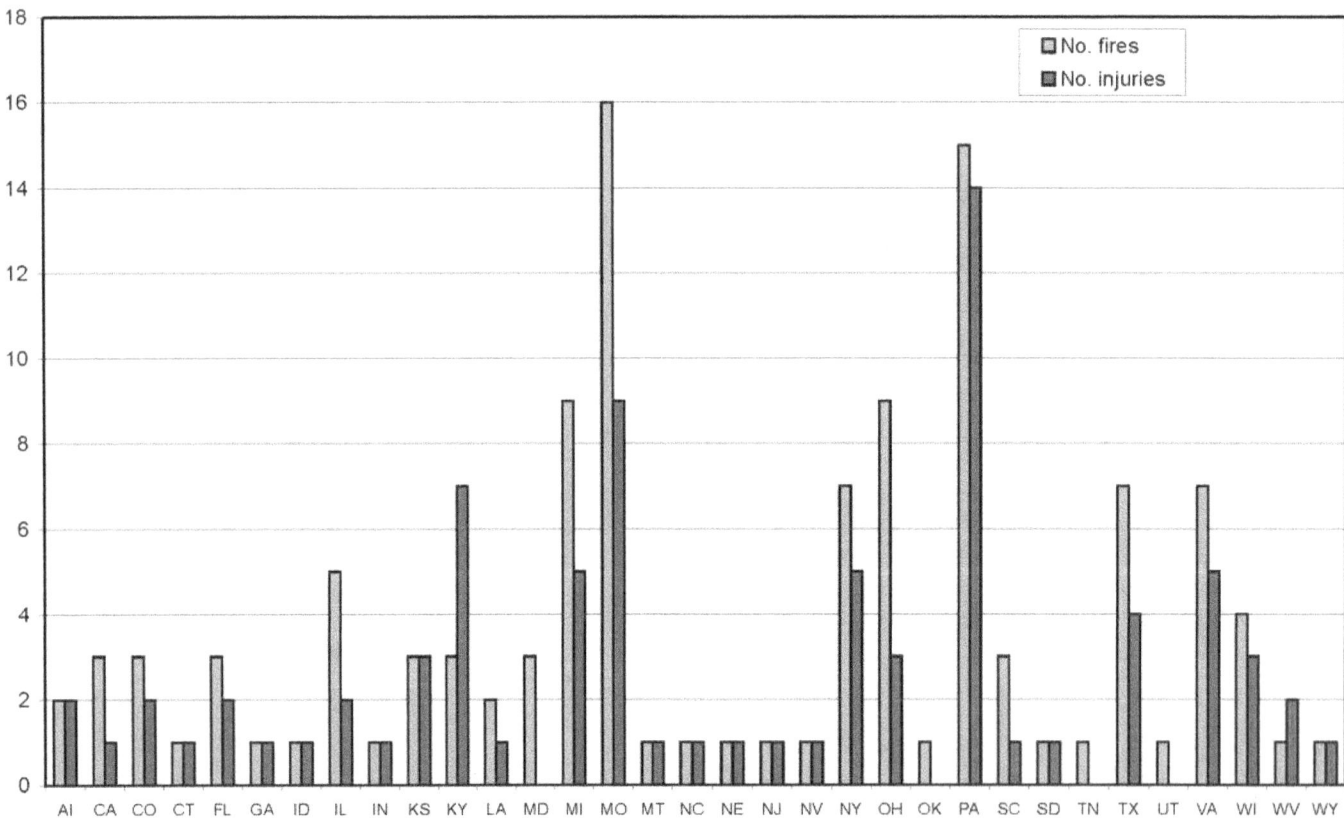

Figure 19.—Number of fires and fire injuries for stone mills by state, 1990–2001.

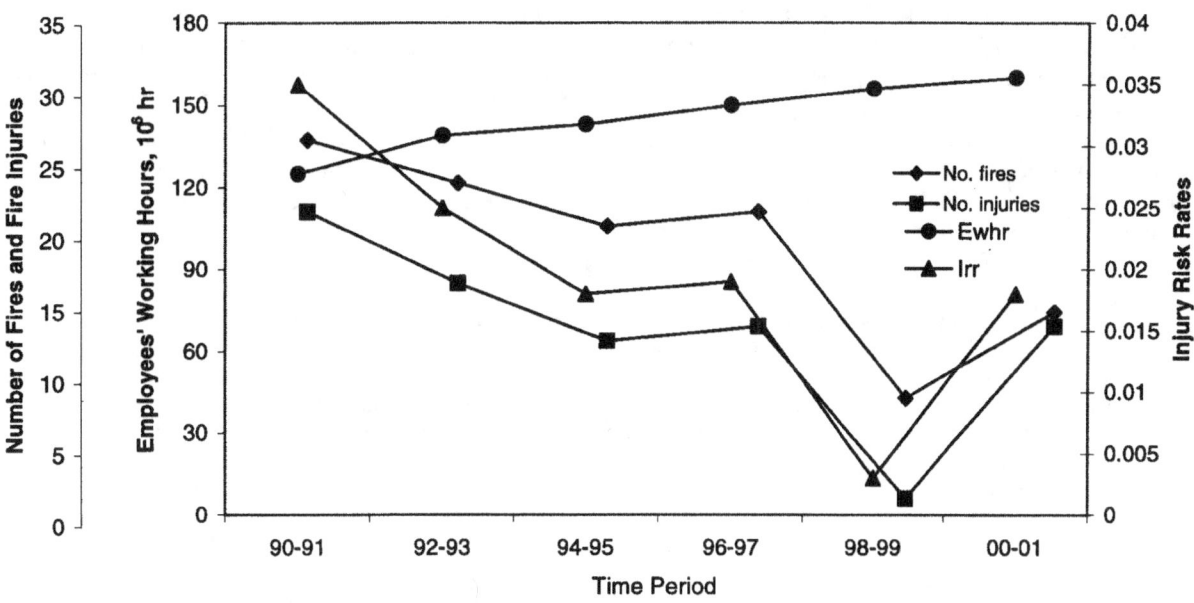

Figure 20.—Number of fires, fire injuries, risk rates, and employees' working hours for stone mills by time period, 1990–2001.

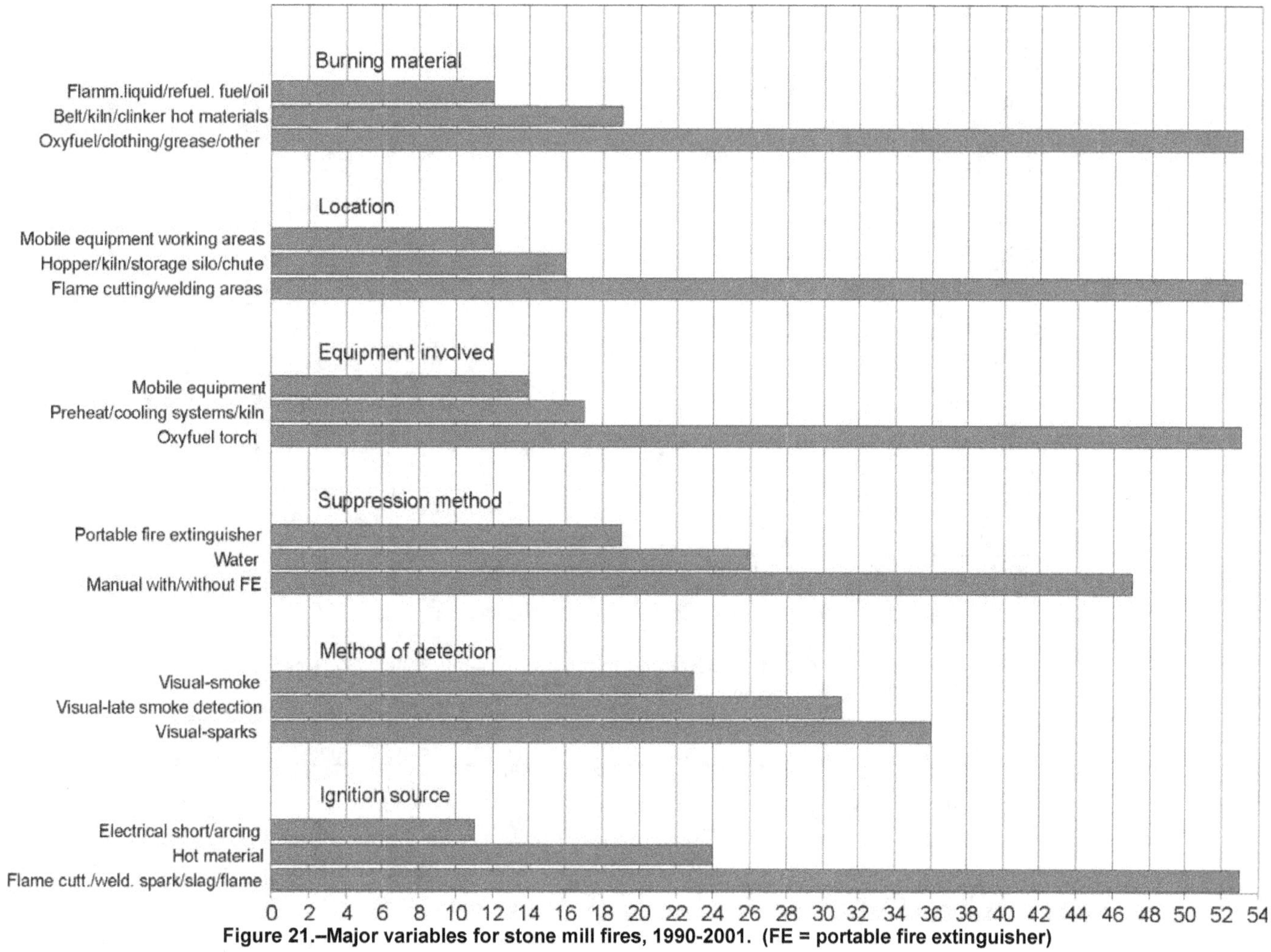

Figure 21.–Major variables for stone mill fires, 1990-2001. (FE = portable fire extinguisher)

equipment involved, and location for 1990–2001. Overall, there were 82 injuries caused by 76 fires. The greatest number of fire injuries occurred in 1990 (15 injuries caused by 15 fires). The ignition sources that caused most of the fire injuries were flame cutting/welding spark/slag/flame, hot material, and flammable liquid/refueling fuel on hot surfaces. Other ignition sources were heat source, hydraulic fluid/fuel sprayed onto equipment hot surfaces, mechanical friction, and electrical short/arcing. The equipment involved in fire injuries included oxyfuel torches, kilns, beltlines, chutes, refueling pumps, and maintenance equipment. Other equipment included heaters, mobile equipment, maintenance equipment, kiln, and electrical systems. The locations where the fire injuries occurred were flame cutting/welding areas, beltlines, kiln and chute areas, and maintenance areas, followed by mobile equipment working areas and transportation areas. Other fire locations were pump stations and beltline areas.

Table 55.—Number of fires, fire injuries, and risk rates for stone mills by state, employees' working hours, and lost workdays, 1990–2001

State[1]	No. fires[1]	No. fire injuries[1]	LWD[2]	Ewhr,[2] 10^6 hr	Irr[3]
Alabama	2	2	249	38.4	0.01
California	3	1	10	38.6	0.005
Colorado	3	2	58	8.5	0.047
Connecticut	1	1	4	5.2	0.039
Florida	2	2	56	28.6	0.014
Georgia	1	1	10	31.2	0.006
Idaho	1	1	13	2.2	0.091
Illinois	5	2	63	36.5	0.011
Indiana	1	1	—	27.6	0.007
Kansas	3	3	104	13.5	0.044
Kentucky	3	7	158	24	0.058
Louisiana	2	1	102	1.1	0.182
Maryland	3	—	—	17	—
Michigan	9	5	95	20.2	0.05
Missouri	16	9	155	56	0.032
Montana	1	1	16	3.7	0.054
Nebraska	1	1	39	5.9	0.034
Nevada	1	1	20	6	0.033
New Jersey	1	1	27	8	0.025
New York	7	5	4	25.5	0.039
North Carolina	1	1	48	23.7	0.008
Ohio	9	3	58	35	0.017
Oklahoma	1	—	—	15.6	—
Pennsylvania	15	14	218	67	0.042
South Carolina	3	1	14	16.2	0.012
South Dakota	1	1	16	5.7	0.035
Tennessee	1	—	66	21.4	—
Texas	7	4	24	54	0.015
Utah	1	—	—	5.2	0.03
Virginia	7	5	153	11	0.091
West Virginia	1	2	90	13.1	0.031
Wisconsin	4	3	41	11	0.055
Wyoming	1	1	—	10	0.02
All other states	—	—	—	186	—
Total	118	82	1,911	873	[3]0.019

[1]Derived from MSHA "Fire Accident Abstract" internal publications.
[2]Derived from MSHA "Injury Experience in Mining" publications.
[3]Calculated according to MSHA formula reported in the "Methodologies" section.

Table 56.—Number of fires, fire injuries, and risk rates for stone mills by time period, employees' working hours, and lost workdays, 1990–2001

	Time period						
	90-91	92-93	94-95	96-97	98-99	00-01	1990-2001
Number of fires[1]	27	24	21	22	9	15	118
Number of fire injuries[1]	22	17	13	14	2	14	82
LWD[2]	377	298	310	388	280	258	1,911
Ewhr,[2] 10^6 hr	125	139	143	150	156	160	873
Irr[3]	0.035	0.024	0.018	0.019	0.003	0.018	[3]0.019

[1]Derived from MSHA "Fire Accident Abstract" internal publications.
[2]Derived from MSHA "Injury Experience in Mining" publications.
[3]Calculated according to MSHA formula reported in the "Methodologies" section.

Table 57.—Number of fires for stone mills by ignition source and time period, 1990–2001

Ignition source	Time period						
	90-91 No. fires	92-93 No. fires	94-95 No. fires	96-97 No. fires	98-99 No. fires	00-01 No. fires	1990-2001 No. fires
Flame cutting/welding spark/slag/flame[1]	14	13	6	14	2	4	53
Hot material	1	5	7	3	3	5	24
Electrical short/arcing	4	2	2	—	3	—	11
Heat source	3	2	1	1	—	2	9
Refueling fuel/flammable liquid/gas on hot surfaces/ collision	2	2	1	1	1	2	9
Hydraulic fluid/fuel on equipment hot surfaces	3	—	1	1	—	1	6
Conveyor belt friction	—	—	1	1	—	—	3
Overheated oil	—	—	1	1	—	—	2
Unknown	—	—	1	—	—	—	1
Total	27	24	21	22	9	15	118

[1]This source caused explosions of pressurized cans and oxyfuel.

Table 58.—Number of fires for stone mills by method of detection and time period, 1990–2001

Method of detection	Time period						
	90-91 No. fires	92-93 No. fires	94-95 No. fires	96-97 No. fires	98-99 No. fires	00-01 No. fires	1990-2001 No. fires
Visual:							
Sparks	9	9	4	10	1	3	36
Smoke	5	2	4	6	2	4	23
Late smoke detection	3	8	7	5	6	2	31
Flames/flash fires	7	2	2	1	—	5	17
Smoldering fire/glow	—	—	1	—	—	1	1
Heard an explosion	2	1	—	—	—	—	3
Undetected	1	2	3	—	—	—	6
Total	27	24	21	22	9	15	118

Table 59.—Number of fires for stone mills by suppression method and time period, 1990–2001

Suppression method	Time period						
	90-91 No. fires	92-93 No. fires	94-95 No. fires	96-97 No. fires	98-99 No. fires	00-01 No. fires	1990-2001 No. fires
Manual with or without FE[1]	12	12	6	12	2	3	47
Water	3	5	6	5	3	4	26
FE	6	3	3	2	2	3	19
FE-foam-DCP-water[2]	4	3	3	3	1	4	18
FSS-foam-water	1	—	—	—	—	—	1
Destroyed/HD[3]	1	1	3	—	1	1	7
Total	27	24	21	22	9	15	118

DCP   Dry chemical powder.
FE   Portable fire extinguisher.
FSS   Machine fire suppression system.
HD Heavily damaged.
[1]Method used by welders to extinguish clothing and oxyfuel/grease fires.
[2]In two instances, fire emergency foam suppression systems were used.
[3]Usually due to failure of firefighting methods, late fire detection, undetected fires, or fire size.

Table 60.—Number of fires for stone mills by equipment involved and time period, 1990–2001

Equipment	Time period						
	90-91 No. fires	92-93 No. fires	94-95 No. fires	96-97 No. fires	98-99 No. fires	00-01 No. fires	1990-2001 No. fires
Oxyfuel torch[1]	14	13	6	14	2	4	53
Kiln/preheat/cooling systems	—	4	5	2	2	4	17
Mobile equipment[2]	5	1	3	3	—	2	14
Electrical system	3	2	2	—	3	—	10
Heater/barrel/refueling pump	3	1	1	1	—	1	7
Beltline	—	1	1	2	1	1	6
Chute/crusher/waste fuel tank/bin feeder/dust collector	1	1	2	—	1	1	6
Facility[3]	—	—	1	—	—	—	1
Maintenance equipment	1	1	—	—	—	—	2
Other	—	—	—	—	—	2	2
Total	27	24	21	22	9	15	118

[1]At times, electrical arc welding equipment was used.
[2]Includes loaders, trucks, drills, and locomotives.
[3]Considered equipment in this report.

Table 61.—Number of fires for stone mills by location and time period, 1990–2001

Location	Time period						
	90-91 No. fires	92-93 No. fires	94-95 No. fires	96-97 No. fires	98-99 No. fires	00-01 No. fires	1990-2001 No. fires
Flame cutting/welding areas[1]	14	13	6	14	2	4	53
Kiln/chute/hopper/silo areas	—	3	6	1	1	5	16
Mobile equipment working areas[2]	4	—	3	3	1	1	12
Beltline areas	—	2	1	2	3	2	10
Maintenance areas/pump station	3	3	1	—	—	1	8
Preheat/cooling areas/bagging station/pit/bin/waste fuel areas	—	2	2	1	1	1	7
Electrical control room/shop/substation	4	—	1	—	1	—	6
Dust collector/chute/crusher areas	1	1	—	1	—	1	4
Facility areas	1	—	1	—	—	—	2
Total	27	24	21	22	9	15	118

[1]Includes hopper, crusher, elevator shaft, chute and kiln areas, and maintenance areas.
[2]Includes pumping station, shop and crusher areas, drilling, loading, haulage, transportation, and fuel preparation areas.

Table 62.—Number of fires for stone mills by burning material and time period, 1990–2001

Burning material	Time period						
	90-91 No. fires	92-93 No. fires	94-95 No. fires	96-97 No. fires	98-99 No. fires	00-01 No. fires	1990-2001 No. fires
Oxyfuel/clothing/grease/other[1]	14	13	6	14	2	4	53
Belt/kiln/clinker hot materials	—	4	6	3	3	3	19
Flammable liquid/oil/refueling fuel	3	3	1	1	—	4	12
Rubber tires/refuse/waste fuel	2	1	3	3	1	1	11
Electrical wires/cables/transformer/battery	4	2	1	—	3	1	11
Hydraulic fluid/fuel	3	—	1	1	—	1	6
Chute/dust collector liners/hopper	—	1	2	—	—	1	4
Facility/content	1	—	1	—	—	—	2
Total	27	24	21	22	9	15	118

[1]Includes rubber hoses, pipelines, dust collector and chute liners, and kiln and shaft materials.

SUMMARY OF MAJOR FIRE AND FIRE INJURY FINDINGS FOR ALL METAL/NONMETAL MINING CATEGORIES

The major fire and fire injury findings for all metal/nonmetal mining categories for 1990–2001 are shown in tables 64–65. Table 66, partly illustrated in figure 22, shows the number of fires, fire injuries, fire fatalities, risk rates, employees' working hours, and lost workdays for all metal/nonmetal mining categories by time period.

For all metal/nonmetal operations (including stone and sand and gravel), a total of 518 fires occurred during 1990–2001; 296 of those fires caused 308 injuries and 4 fatalities (Ewhr = 4,012 × 10^6 hr, Irr = 0.015, LWD = 36,204). Thirty fires and 26 injuries involved contractors. The greatest number of fires and fire injuries occurred at surface operations; the highest risk rate values were also calculated for surface operations. The number of fires increased during the first four 2-year time periods (1990–1991, 1992–1993, 1994–1995, and 1996–1997), then decreased during the last two periods (1998–1999 and 2000–2001). The number of injuries showed a decrease throughout the periods, accompanied by an increase in employees' working hours.

Twenty-five firefighting interventions by mine rescue teams in underground mines and at least 30 interventions at surface operations were required to combat these fires. However, 45 fires destroyed or heavily damaged facilities and equipment (including 19 pieces of mobile equipment) because of failure of firefighting methods, late fire detection, undetected fires, or fire

size. Ninety-seven fires were detected late, and 30 fires were undetected.

The ignition sources that caused the greatest number of fires were flame cutting/welding spark/slag/flame (169 fires or 33% with 137 injuries), hydraulic fluid/fuel sprayed onto equipment hot surfaces (89 fires or 17% with 46 injuries and 3 fatalities), heat source/explosion and flammable liquids/ gas/refueling fuel on hot surfaces (98 fires or 19% with 73 injuries), electrical short/arcing (51 fires or 10% with 16 injuries), and spontaneous combustion/hot material (46 fires or 9% with 17 injuries).

The flame cutting/welding spark/slag/flame source caused fires usually involving welders' clothing or oxyfuel/grease and other materials (including chute and dust collector liners, flammable liquids, belt material, crusher, hopper and shaker deck materials, washer plants, equipment mechanical components, stampler breaker, hydraulic fluid, rubber tires and hoses, gear boxes, bin feeder, dump rope cables, screen liner and screen panel, kiln and shaft material, pipelines, liquor pumps, wood pallets, electrical junction boxes, handrails, grease, refuse, shop and wood). The spontaneous combustion/hot material and electrical fires were usually detected late due to lack of combustion gas/smoke detection systems. At least 55 of the 89 mobile equipment hydraulic fluid/fuel fires became large fires (requiring 12 mine rescue team interventions in underground mines and at least 6 interventions at surface operations) because of the continuous flow of fluid/fuel from the pumps due to engine shutoff failure, lack of an emergency hydraulic line drainage system, difficulty in activating available emergency systems at the ground level, or lack of effective and rapid local firefighting response capabilities. Ten pieces of mobile equipment involved in fires had machine fire suppression systems. Dual activations (two activations) of machine fire suppression and engine shutoff systems succeeded in temporarily abating the fires, which reignited, fueled by the flow of pressurized fluids entrapped in the lines. In at least 13 instances the cab was suddenly engulfed in flames, forcing the operators to make an unsafe exit, probably due to the ignition of flammable vapors and mists that penetrated the cab. Of note is that the hydraulic fluid fires subsequently involved the fuel system.

The major findings for each metal/nonmetal mining category are discussed below.

1. In underground metal/nonmetal and stone mines, 65 fires occurred; 6 of the fires caused 9 injuries (Ewhr = 260×10^6 hr, Irr = 0.007, LWD = 83). The leading ignition sources were hydraulic fluid/fuel sprayed onto equipment hot surfaces

(16 fires or 25%), flame cutting/welding spark/slag/flame (13 fires or 20%), and electrical short/arcing (12 fires or 19%). The flame cutting/welding spark/slag/flame source caused fires involving oxyfuel/clothing/grease and other materials (including rubber tires and hoses, hydraulic fluid, shop, refuse, wood, chute liner, and shaft material). The electrical fires were usually detected long after the fires had started due to lack of combustion gas/smoke detection systems. Thirteen of the 16 mobile equipment hydraulic fluid/fuel fires became large fires (requiring 12 mine rescue team interventions) because of the continuous flow of fluids from the pumps due to engine shutoff failure, lack of an emergency hydraulic line drainage system, difficulty in activating available emergency systems at ground level, or lack of effective and rapid local firefighting response capabilities. In two instances during these fires, the cab was suddenly engulfed in flames, probably due to the ignition of flammable vapors and mists that penetrated the cab. Four pieces of equipment involved in fires had machine fire suppression systems. Dual activations (two activations) of machine fire suppression and engine shutoff systems succeeded in temporarily abating the fires; however, the flames reignited, fueled by the pressurized fluids entrapped in the lines.

Table 63.—Number of fire injuries per number of fires causing injuries and total fires for stone mills by year, ignition source, equipment involved, and location, 1990–2001

Year	No. total fires	No. fires causing injuries	No. fire injuries	Ignition source	Equipment	Location
1990	19	15	11	Flame cutting/welding spark/slag/flame	Oxyfuel torch	Flame cutting/welding areas.[1]
			1	Heat source	Heater	Maintenance area.
			1	Flammable liquid on hot surfaces	Refueling pump	Pump station.
			2	Hydraulic fluid/fuel on equipment hot surfaces	Truck	Haulage area.
1991	8	6	2	Flame cutting/welding spark/slag/flame	Oxyfuel torch	Flame cutting/welding areas.[1]
			1	Heat source	Heater	Maintenance area.
			2	Flammable liquid on hot surfaces	Maintenance equipment	Maintenance area.
			1	Hydraulic fluid/fuel on equipment hot surfaces	Loader	Loading area.
			1	Electrical short/arcing	Locomotive	Transportation area.
1992	10	7	5	Flame cutting/welding spark/slag/flame	Oxyfuel torch	Flame cutting/welding areas.[1]
			1	Hot material	Chute	Chute area.
			1	Heat source	Heater	Hopper area.
1993	14	10	6	Flame cutting/welding spark/slag/flame	Oxyfuel torch	Flame cutting/welding areas.[1]
			2	Flammable liquid on hot surfaces	Maintenance equipment	Maintenance area.
			1	Hot material	Preheat system	Preheat tower.
			1	Heat source	Heater	Maintenance area.
1994	9	8	6	Flame cutting/welding spark/slag/flame	Oxyfuel torch	Flame cutting/welding areas.[1]
			1	Hot material	Beltline	Beltline areas.
			1	Hydraulic fluid/fuel on equipment hot surfaces	Truck	Haulage area.
1995	12	5	1	Electrical short/arcing	Electrical system	Electrical control room.
			2	Hot material	Hopper/kiln-chute	Hopper/kiln chute/loading areas.
			1	Refueling fuel on hot surfaces	Kiln	Kiln area.
			1	Heat source	Heater	Maintenance area.
1996	14	10	9	Flame cutting/welding spark/slag/flame	Oxyfuel torch	Flame cutting/welding areas.[1]
			1	Hydraulic fluid/fuel on equipment hot surfaces	Truck	Haulage area.
1997	8	4	4	Flame cutting/welding spark/slag/flame	Oxyfuel torch	Flame cutting/welding areas.[1]
1998	6	—	—	—	—	—
1999	3	2	2	Flame cutting/welding spark/slag/flame	Oxyfuel torch	Flame cutting/welding areas.[1]
2000	6	4	3	Flame cutting/welding spark/slag/flame	Oxyfuel torch	Flame cutting/welding areas.[1]
			1	Mechanical friction	Kiln	Kiln area.
2001	9	5	2	Refueling fuel on hot surfaces	Kiln	Kiln area.
			1	Flame cutting/welding spark/slag/flame	Oxyfuel torch	Flame cutting/welding areas.[1]
			6	Hot material	Beltline	Kiln/beltline areas.
			1	Heat source	Heater	Maintenance area.
Total	118	76	82			

[1]Includes hopper, shaft, piping, chute and kiln areas, and mobile equipment maintenance areas.

Table 64.—Major fire findings for all metal/nonmetal mining categories, 1990–2001

Variables	Underground metal/nonmetal and stone mines	Surface of underground metal/nonmetal and stone mines	Surface metal/nonmetal mines	Surface sand and gravel mines	Surface stone mines	Metal/nonmetal mills	Stone mills
GT: No. fires: 519 No. fires causing injuries: 296 LWD: 36,204	No. fires: 65 No. fires causing injuries: 6 LWD: 83	No. fires: 12 No. fires causing injuries: 5 LWD: 75	No. fires: 79 No. fires causing injuries: 45 LWD: 13,134	No. fires: 71 No. fires causing injuries: 59 LWD: 6,921	No. fires: 97 No. fires causing injuries: 68 LWD: 7,399	No. fires: 77 No. fires causing injuries: 37 LWD: 6,681	No. fires: 118 No. fires causing injuries: 76 LWD: 1,911
Ignition source	Hydraulic fluid/fuel on equipment hot surfaces Flame cutting/welding spark/slag/flame Electrical short/arcing	Flame cutting/welding spark/slag/flame Electrical short/arcing Heat source	Hydraulic fluid/fuel on equipment hot surfaces Flame cutting/welding spark/slag/flame Electrical short/arcing	Flame cutting/welding spark/slag/flame Heat source Hydraulic fluid/fuel on equipment hot surfaces	Flame cutting/welding spark/slag/flame Heat source-flammable liquid Hydraulic fluid/fuel on equipment hot surfaces	Flame cutting/welding spark/slag/flame Spontaneous combustion/hot material Electrical short/arcing	Flame cutting/welding spark/slag/flame Hot material/spontaneous combustion Electrical short/arcing
Method of detection	Visual-late smoke detection Visual-flames/flash fires Visual-smoke	Visual-sparks Visual-smoke/fumes Visual-late smoke detection	Visual-flames/flash fires Visual-smoke Visual-sparks	Visual-flames/flash fires Visual-sparks Visual-smoke	Visual-flames/flash fires Visual-sparks Visual-smoke	Visual-late smoke detection Visual-sparks Visual-flames/flash fires	Visual-sparks Visual-late smoke detection Visual-smoke Visual flames/flash fire
Suppression method	FE-DCP/foam/water Water FE	Water Manual with or without FE FE	FE-foam/DCP/water FE Manual with or without FE	Manual/FE FE-foam/DCP/water Water	Manual with or without FE Water FE-DCP/foam/water	Water FE Manual with or without FE	Manual with or without FE Water FE
Equipment	Mobile equipment[1] Oxyfuel torch Beltline/drive/pulley	Oxyfuel torch Facilities Heater	Mobile equipment[1] Oxyfuel torch Heater	Oxyfuel torch Mobile equipment[1] Heater/burner	Mobile equipment[1] Heater/maintenance equipment/burner Oxyfuel torch	Oxyfuel torch Dust collector/other Pump/oil vaporizer	Oxyfuel torch Kiln/preheat/cooling system Mobile equipment[1] Electrical system
Location	Mobile equipment working areas[2] Flame cutting/welding areas[3] Mine face/other areas	Flame cutting/welding areas[3] Facility/garage/other Fan housing	Mobile equipment working areas[2] Flame cutting/welding areas[3] Maintenance areas/other	Flame cutting/welding areas[3] Maintenance areas Mobile equipment working areas[2]	Maintenance areas/other Flame cutting/welding areas[3] Mobile equipment working areas[2]	Flame cutting/welding areas[3] Dust collector/other areas Maintenance areas	Flame cutting/welding areas[3] Kiln/other areas Kiln/chute/hopper/silo Mobile equipment working areas[2]
Burning material	Hydraulic fluid Oxyfuel/clothing/grease/other Electrical cord/wire/cable/battery	Oxyfuel/clothing/grease/other Facility/content Wood	Hydraulic fluid/fuel/oil Oxyfuel/clothing/grease/other Flammable liquid/material	Oxyfuel/clothing/grease/other Hydraulic fluid/fuel Flammable liquid/gas	Oxyfuel/clothing/grease/other Hazardous material/chemical/other Hydraulic fluid/fuel	Oxyfuel/clothing/grease/other Belt material Flammable liquid/refueling fuel	Oxyfuel/clothing/grease/other Belt/kiln/clinker hot materials Flammable liquid/refueling fuel/oil

DCP Dry chemical powder.   FE Portable fire extinguisher.   GT Grand total.

[1]Includes golf and ore carts, locomotives, loaders, scoops, shuttle cars, power scalers, trolleys, trucks, drills, dozers, shovels, scrapers, dredges, buckets, tankers, and forklifts.

[2]Includes haulage, loading, mucking, decline slopes, panel and tunnel areas, transportation, drilling, mining, excavating areas, pumping stations, shop and crusher areas, fuel preparation and dredging areas.

[3]Includes shops, mainways, boreholes, shafts, stations, slusher bucket, chute, dust collector, hopper, crusher and kiln areas, junction boxes, facilities and shops, head frame, walkways, pipeline, dump rope, crowd platform, storage bin, baghouse, pelletizer building, liquor pump, beltline, generator housing, deck and bin feeder, stampler breaker and screen shaft and compactor areas, and washer plants.

NOTE.—Variables are listed in descending order of occurrence.

47

Table 65.—Major fire injury findings for all metal/nonmetal mining categories, 1990–2001

Variables	Underground metal/nonmetal and stone mines	Surface of underground metal/nonmetal and stone mines	Surface metal/nonmetal mines	Surface sand and gravel mines	Surface stone mines	Metal/nonmetal mills	Stone mills
GT: No. fire injuries:	308	9	44	60	67	41	82
No. fire fatalities:	4		2		1	1	
Ewhr, 10^6 hr:	4,012	260	546	741	689	845	873
Irr:	0.015	0.007	0.016	0.016	0.02	0.01	0.019
Ignition source	Hydraulic fluid/fuel on equipment hot surfaces; Flame cutting/welding spark/slag/flame; Overheated oil on hot surfaces	Flame cutting/welding spark/slag/flame	Hydraulic fluid/fuel on equipment hot surfaces; Flame cutting/welding spark/slag/flame; Flammable liquid/refueling fuel/oil on hot surfaces	Flame cutting/welding spark/slag/flame; Heat source; Hydraulic fluid/fuel on equipment hot surfaces	Flame cutting/welding spark/slag/flame; Heat source; Hydraulic fluid/fuel on equipment hot surfaces	Flame cutting/welding spark/slag/flame; Flammable liquid/refueling fuel on hot surfaces/explosion; Hot materials	Flame cutting/welding spark/slag/flame; Hot material; Flammable liquid/gas/refueling fuel on hot surfaces
Method of detection	Visual-flames/flash fires; Visual-sparks; Visual-smoke	Visual-sparks	Visual-flames/flash fires; Visual-sparks; Visual-smoke	Visual-sparks; Visual-smoke; Visual-flames/flash fires	Visual-sparks; Visual-smoke; Visual flames/flash fires	Visual-sparks; Visual-flames; Visual-late smoke detection	Visual-sparks; Visual-smoke; Visual-flames
Suppression method	FE-DCP/foam/water; Manual with or without FE; FE	Manual with or without FE	FE-foam/DCP/water; Manual with or without FE; FE	Manual with or without FE; Water; FE-foam/DCP/water	Manual with or without FE; FE; FE-foam/DCP/water	Manual with or without FE; FE; Water	Manual with or without FE; Water; FE
Equipment	Mobile equipment; Oxyfuel torch; Air compressors/mobile equipment	Oxyfuel torch	Mobile equipment; Oxyfuel torch; Maintenance equipment/mobile equipment	Oxyfuel torch; Heater; Mobile equipment	Oxyfuel torch; Heater; Mobile equipment	Oxyfuel torch; Maintenance equipment/liquor pump; Product cooling system	Oxyfuel torch; Beltline/chute/kiln/preheat system; Maintenance equipment/refueling pump/mobile equipment
Location	Mobile equipment working areas; Flame cutting/welding areas; Mine face/panel section	Flame cutting/welding area	Mobile equipment working areas; Flame cutting/welding areas; Maintenance areas	Flame cutting/welding areas; Maintenance/refuse/beltline areas; Mobile equipment working areas	Flame cutting/welding areas; Beltline/maintenance/working areas; Mobile equipment working areas	Flame cutting/welding areas; Maintenance/liquor/pump/refinery areas; Product cooler area	Flame cutting/welding areas; Preheat/kiln/chute/beltline areas; Maintenance areas/pump station
Burning material	Hydraulic fluid/fuel; Oxyfuel/clothing/grease/other; Oil	Oxyfuel/clothing/grease/other	Hydraulic fluid/fuel; Oxyfuel/clothing/grease/other; Flammable liquid/refueling fuel/oil	Oxyfuel/clothing/grease/other; Refuse; Hydraulic fluid/fuel	Oxyfuel/clothing/grease/other; Refuse/hazardous material; Hydraulic fluid/fuel	Oxyfuel/clothing/grease; Flammable liquid/refueling fuel; Material/belt	Oxyfuel/clothing/grease/other; Material/belt; Flammable liquid/gas/refueling fuel

DCP Dry chemical powder.
FE Portable fire extinguisher.
GT Grand total.
NOTE.—Variables are listed in descending order of occurrence.

48

Table 66.—Number of fires, fire injuries, fire fatalities, and risk rates for all metal/nonmetal mining categories
by time period, employees' working hours, and lost workdays, 1990–2001

	Time period						1990-2001
	90-91	92-93	94-95	96-97	98-99	00-01	
Number of fires[1]	92	115	100	93	54	64	518
Number of fire injuries[1]	62	69	61	53	28	35	308
Number of fire fatalities[1]	—	1	2	—	—	1	4
LWD[2]	941	7,014	13,510	6,864	1,026	6,849	36,204
Ewhr,[2] 10^6 hr	652	650	664	681	677	688	4,012
Irr[3]	0.019	0.02	0.018	0.016	0.008	0.01	[3]0.015

[1]Derived from MSHA "Fire Accident Abstract" internal publications.
[2]Derived from MSHA "Injury Experience in Mining" publications.
[3]Calculated according to MSHA formula reported in the "Methodologies" section.

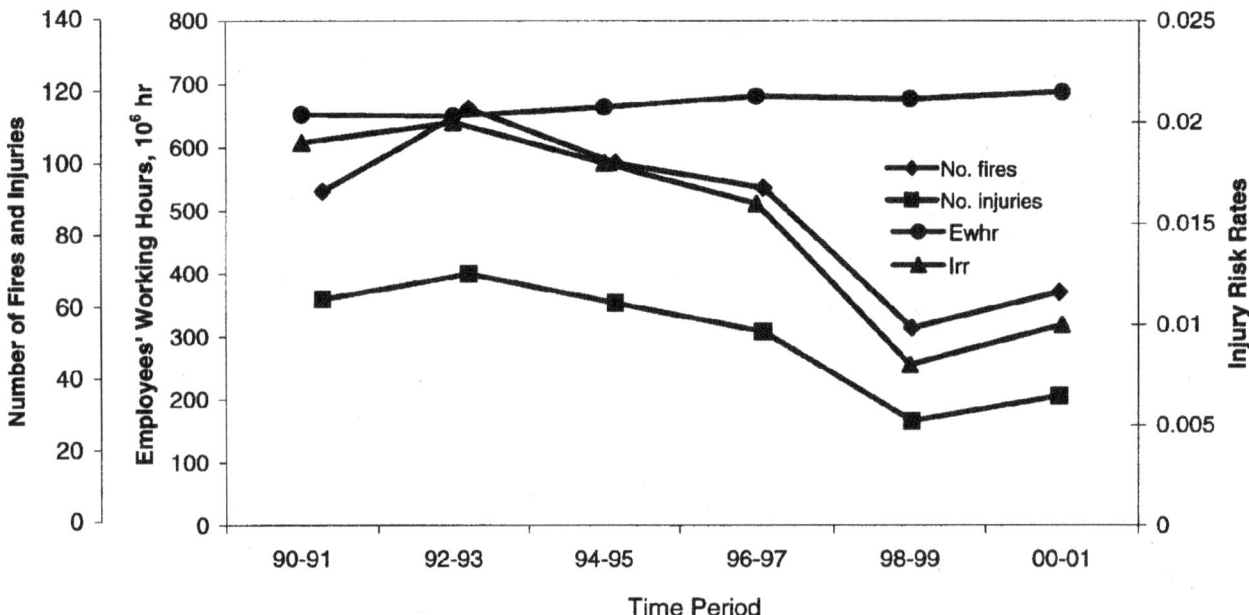

Figure 22.—Number of fires, fire injuries, risk rates, and employees' working hours for all metal/nonmetal mining categories
by time period, 1990–2001.

Upon mine/section evacuation (required 30 times), mine rescue teams (required 25 times), often hindered by dense smoke in reaching the fire location, fought the fires (including 12 mobile equipment fires) with dry chemical powder, rock dust, and water; in one instance, foam was also used. However, five fires destroyed or heavily damaged equipment (including four pieces of mobile equipment) because of failure of firefighting methods, late fire detection, undetected fires, or fire size. Eighteen fires were detected late, and two were undetected.

The ignition sources that caused the underground fire injuries were hydraulic fluid/fuel sprayed onto equipment hot surfaces, flame cutting/welding spark/slag/flame, and overheated oil. The equipment involved in fire injuries included mobile equipment, oxyfuel torches, and air compressors. The locations where fire injuries occurred were mobile equipment working areas, flame cutting/welding areas, and mine face and panel section.

2. At surface of underground metal/nonmetal and stone mines, 12 fires occurred; 5 of the fires caused 5 injuries (Ewhr = 58 × 10^6 hr, Irr = 0.017, LWD = 75). The leading ignition source was flame cutting/welding spark/slag/flame (7 fires or 58%), followed by electrical short/arcing and heat source. The flame cutting/welding spark/slag/flame source caused fires involving oxyfuel/clothing/grease and other materials (including electrical junction boxes, handrails, grease, flammable liquids, rubber tires, and equipment mechanical components). In all, three fires destroyed or heavily damaged equipment. Two fires were detected late, and three fires were undetected. The ignition source that caused the fire injuries was flame cutting/welding spark/slag/flame.

3. At surface metal/nonmetal mines, 79 fires occurred; 45 of the fires caused 44 injuries and 2 fatalities (Ewhr = 546 × 10^6 hr, Irr = 0.016, LWD = 13,134). The leading ignition source was hydraulic fluid/fuel sprayed onto equipment hot surfaces (35 fires or 44%), followed by flame cutting/welding spark/slag/flame (13 fires or 17%) and electrical short/arcing (8 fires or 10%). The flame cutting/welding spark/slag/flame source caused fires involving oxyfuel/clothing/grease and other

materials (involving rubber hoses, grease, equipment mechanical components, dump rope cables, screen liner, and shaft materials). Twenty-two of the 35 mobile equipment hydraulic fluid/ fuel fires became large fires because of the continuous flow of fluid/fuel from the pumps due to engine shutoff failure, lack of an emergency line drainage system, difficulty in activating available emergency systems at ground level, or lack of effective and rapid local firefighting response capabilities. In at least five instances the cab was suddenly engulfed in flames, probably due to the ignition of flammable vapors and mists that penetrated the cabs. Five pieces of mobile equipment involved in fires had machine fire suppression systems. Dual activation (one activation) of machine fire suppression and engine shutoff systems succeeded in temporarily abating the fires; however, the flames reignited, fueled by the flow of fluids entrapped in the lines.

In at least five instances, including one mobile equipment fire, fire brigades and fire departments fought the fires with foam, dry chemical powder, and water. However, nine fires destroyed or heavily damaged equipment (including seven pieces of mobile equipment) because of failure of firefighting methods, late fire detection, undetected fires, or fire size. Eight fires were detected late, and three fires were undetected.

The ignition sources that caused most of the fire injuries were hydraulic fluid/fuel sprayed onto equipment hot surfaces, flame cutting/welding spark/slag/flame, and flammable liquid/refueling fuel/oil on hot surfaces. The equipment most often involved in fire injuries included mobile equipment, oxyfuel torches, and maintenance equipment. The locations where most of the fire injuries occurred were mobile equipment working areas, flame cutting/ welding areas, and maintenance areas.

4. At surface sand and gravel mines, 70 fires occurred; 59 of the fires caused 60 injuries (Ewhr = 741 × 10⁶ hr, Irr = 0.016, LWD = 6,921). The leading ignition sources were flame cutting/ welding spark/slag/flame (29 fires or 41%), heat source/ explosion (15 fires or 21%), and hydraulic fluid/fuel sprayed onto equipment hot surfaces (14 fires or 20%). The flame cutting/welding spark/ slag/flame source caused fires involving oxyfuel/clothing/ grease and other materials (including chute liners, washer plant, crusher, hopper and shaker deck, flammable liquids, equipment mechanical components, and belt materials). Five of the 14 mobile equipment hydraulic fluid/fuel fires became large fires because of the continuous flow of fluid/fuel from the pumps due to engine shutoff failure, lack of an emergency line drainage system, difficulty in activating available emergency systems at ground level, or lack of effective and rapid local fire response capabilities. In two instances the cab was suddenly engulfed in flames, probably due to the ignition of flammable vapors and mists that penetrated the cab. None of the equipment involved in fires had machine fire suppression systems.

On at least three occasions, including one mobile equipment fire, fire brigades and fire departments fought the fires with foam, dry chemical powder, and water. However, four fires destroyed or heavily damaged equipment (including two pieces of mobile equipment) because of failure of firefighting methods, late fire detection, undetected fires, or fire size. Eight fires were detected late, and four fires were undetected.

The ignition sources that caused most of the fire injuries were flame cutting/welding spark/slag/flame, heat source, and hydraulic fluid/fuel sprayed onto equipment hot surfaces. The equipment most often involved in fire injuries included oxyfuel torches, heaters, and mobile equipment. The locations where most of the fire injuries occurred were flame cutting/welding areas, maintenance areas, and mobile equipment working areas.

5. At surface stone mines, 97 fires occurred; 68 of the fires caused 67 injuries and 1 fatality (Ewhr = 689 × 10⁶ hr, Irr = 0.02, LWD = 7,399). The leading ignition sources were flame cutting/ welding spark/slag/flame (25 fires or 26%), heat source/explosion-flammable liquid/gas (24 fire or 25%), and hydraulic fluid/fuel sprayed onto equipment hot surfaces (16 fires or 17%). The flame cutting/welding spark/slag/flame source caused fires involving oxyfuel/clothing/grease and other materials (including screen panel and chute liner, crusher and hopper, stampler breaker, rubber hoses, gear boxes, bin feeder, hydraulic fluid, and shaft material). None of the mobile equipment involved in fires had machine fire suppression systems. Ten of the 16 mobile equipment hydraulic fluid/fuel fires became large fires because of the continuous flow of fluid/fuel from the pumps due to engine shutoff failure, lack of an emergency line drainage system, or lack of effective and rapid local firefighting response capabilities. In two instances the cab was suddenly engulfed in flames, probably due to the ignition of flammable vapors and mists that penetrated the cab.

In at least six instances, including one mobile equipment fire, fire brigades and fire departments fought the fires with foam, dry chemical powder, and water. However, 12 fires destroyed or heavily damaged equipment (including four pieces of mobile equipment) because of failure of firefighting methods, late fire detection, undetected fires, or fire size. Four fires were detected late; eight were undetected fires.

The ignition sources that caused most of the fire injuries were flame cutting/welding spark/slag/flame, heat source, and hydraulic fluid/fuel sprayed onto equipment hot surfaces. The equipment most often involved in fire injuries included oxyfuel torches, heaters, and mobile equipment. The locations where most of the fire injuries occurred were flame cutting/welding areas, maintenance areas, refuse and fire pot areas, and mobile equipment working areas.

6. At metal/nonmetal mills, 77 fires occurred; 37 of the fires caused 41 injuries and 1 fatality (Ewhr = 845 × 10⁶ hr, Irr = 0.01, LWD = 6,681). The leading ignition sources were flame cutting/ welding spark/slag/flame (29 fires or 38%), hot material (12 fires or 16%), and flammable liquid/refueling fuel/oil on hot surfaces (9 fires or 12%). The flame cutting/welding spark/ slag/ flame source caused fires involving oxyfuel/clothing/grease and other materials (including liquor pumps, belt material, pipelines, flammable liquids, dust collector and chute liners, wood pallets, crusher, and screen panel). The hot material fires and electrical fires were usually detected long after they had started due to lack of combustion gas/smoke detection systems. One of the three mobile equipment hydraulic fluid/fuel fires became a large pump fire because of the continuous flow of fluid from the pump due

to engine shutoff failure. In this instance the cab was suddenly engulfed in flames, probably due to the ignition of flammable vapors and mists that penetrated the cab.

In at least five instances, including one mobile equipment fire, fire brigades and fire department fought the fires with foam, dry chemical powder, and water. However, six fires destroyed or heavily damaged equipment (including one piece of mobile equipment) because of failure of firefighting methods, late fire detection, undetected fires, or fire size. Twenty-six fires were detected late, and four were undetected.

The ignition sources that caused most of the fire injuries were flame cutting/welding spark/slag/flame, flammable liquids/refueling fuel on hot surfaces/explosion, and hot material. The equipment involved in fire injuries included oxyfuel torches, maintenance equipment, refueling and liquor pumps, and product cooling system. The locations where the fire injuries occurred were flame cutting/welding areas, maintenance areas, pump housing and liquor pump areas, and product cooling area.

7. At stone mills, 118 fires occurred; 76 of the fires caused 82 injuries (Ewhr = 873×10^6 hr, Irr = 0.019, LWD = 1,911). The leading ignition sources were flame cutting/welding spark/slag/flame (53 fires or 45%), hot material (24 fires or 20%), and electrical short/arcing (11 fires or 9%).

The flame cutting/welding spark/slag/flame source caused fires involving oxyfuel/clothing/grease and other materials (including rubber hoses, pipelines, dust collector and chute liners, and shaft and kiln materials). Four of the five hydraulic fluid/fuel fires became large fires because of the continuous flow of fluids from the pumps due to engine shutoff failure, lack of an emergency line drainage system, difficulty in activating emergency systems at ground level, or lack of effective and rapid local firefighting response capabilities. In one instance the cab was suddenly engulfed in flames, probably due to the ignition of flammable vapors and mists that penetrated the cab. Of the six pieces of mobile equipment involved in fires, one had a machine fire suppression system, which, upon activation with the engine shutoff system, succeeded in temporarily abating the fire.

In at least 11 instances, including 2 mobile equipment fires, fire brigades and fire departments fought the fires with foam, dry chemical powder, and water. In two instances, emergency foam fire suppression systems were used. However, seven fires destroyed or heavily damaged equipment (including one piece of mobile equipment) because of failure of firefighting methods. Thirty-one fires were detected late, and six fires were undetected.

The ignition sources that caused most of the fire injuries were flame cutting/welding spark/slag/flame, hot material, and flammable liquid/gas/refueling fuel on hot surfaces. The equipment most often involved in fires included oxyfuel torches, kilns, beltlines, chute, preheat system, and maintenance equipment. Most of the fire injuries occurred at flame cutting/welding areas, kiln, beltline and chute areas, preheat areas, and maintenance areas.

CONCLUSIONS

During 1990–2001, a total of 518 fires occurred in all metal/nonmetal mining categories; 296 of those fires caused 308 injuries and 4 fatalities. Surface operations had the most fires and the highest injury risk rate values. Forty-five fires destroyed or heavily damaged facilities and equipment (including 19 pieces of mobile equipment) because of failure of firefighting methods, late fire detection, undetected fires, or fire size.

In the future, many of these fires and injuries might be prevented or detected and extinguished at their earliest stage by improving current fire safety procedures, adopting existing/improved fire detection and suppression technologies, and/or developing new technologies. Several strategies for reducing and/or preventing the number of fires and fire injuries follow.

1. Increase vigilance, improve safety procedures, and develop new technologies in order to prevent fires and injuries caused by flame cutting and welding operations.

2. Improve equipment hydraulic/fuel/electrical systems inspection programs; adopt fire-resistant hydraulic fluids and electrically powered motors for use in underground mines; develop new technologies (equipment/cab rapid fire detection/prevention/suppression systems, emergency line drainage systems, and fire barriers); adopt an optimal ground level location for the activation of emergency systems; improve operator's fire preparedness training programs; and develop effective and rapid local firefighting response capabilities.

3. Adopt existing/improved systems for continuous and early detection of combustion gases and smoke along beltlines.

4. Adopt existing/improved technologies for monitoring equipment (beltlines) operational functions.

5. Increase vigilance and adopt improved safety procedures for handling flammable liquids and refueling fuel in the vicinity of heat sources.

ACKNOWLEDGMENT

The author thanks Kimberly A. Mitchell, Program Operations Assistant, NIOSH Pittsburgh Research Laboratory, for computerizing the tables and figures in this report.

REFERENCES

Butani SJ, Pomroy WH [1987]. A statistical analysis of metal and nonmetal mine fire incidents in the United States from 1950 to 1984. Minneapolis, MN: U.S. Department of the Interior, Bureau of Mines, Twin Cities Research Center, IC 9132.

CFR. Code of Federal regulations. Washington, DC: U.S. Government Printing Office, Office of the Federal Register.

De Rosa MI [2004]. Analyses of mobile equipment fires for all U.S. surface and underground coal and metal/nonmetal mining categories, 1990–1999. Pittsburgh, PA: U.S. Department of Health and Human Services, Public Health Service, Centers for Disease Control and Prevention, National Institute for Occupational Safety and Health, DHHS (NIOSH) Publication No. 2004–105, IC 9467.

MSHA [1991a]. Injury experience in metallic mineral mining, 1990. Denver, CO: U.S. Department of Labor, Mine Safety and Health Administration, Office of Injury and Employment Information, IR 1201.

MSHA [1991b]. Injury experience in nonmetal mineral mining (except stone and coal), 1990. Denver, CO: U.S. Department of Labor, Mine Safety and Health Administration, Office of Injury and Employment Information, IR 1202.

MSHA [1991c]. Injury experience in sand and gravel mining, 1990. Denver, CO: U.S. Department of Labor, Mine Safety and Health Administration, Office of Injury and Employment Information, IR 1204.

MSHA [1991d]. Injury experience in stone mining, 1990. Denver, CO: U.S. Department of Labor, Mine Safety and Health Administration, Office of Injury and Employment Information, IR 1203.

MSHA [1992a]. Injury experience in metallic mineral mining, 1991. Denver, CO: U.S. Department of Labor, Mine Safety and Health Administration, Office of Injury and Employment Information, IR 1208.

MSHA [1992b]. Injury experience in nonmetal mineral mining (except stone and coal), 1991. Denver, CO: U.S. Department of Labor, Mine Safety and Health Administration, Office of Injury and Employment Information, IR 1209.

MSHA [1992c]. Injury experience in sand and gravel mining, 1991. Denver, CO: U.S. Department of Labor, Mine Safety and Health Administration, Office of Injury and Employment Information, IR 1211.

MSHA [1992d]. Injury experience in stone mining, 1991. Denver, CO: U.S. Department of Labor, Mine Safety and Health Administration, Office of Injury and Employment Information, IR 1210.

MSHA [1993a]. Injury experience in metallic mineral mining, 1992. Denver, CO: U.S. Department of Labor, Mine Safety and Health Administration, Office of Injury and Employment Information, IR 1218.

MSHA [1993b]. Injury experience in nonmetal mineral mining (except stone and coal), 1992. Denver, CO: U.S. Department of Labor, Mine Safety and Health Administration, Office of Injury and Employment Information, IR 1219.

MSHA [1993c]. Injury experience in sand and gravel mining, 1992. Denver, CO: U.S. Department of Labor, Mine Safety and Health Administration, Office of Injury and Employment Information, IR 1217.

MSHA [1993d]. Injury experience in stone mining, 1992. Denver, CO: U.S. Department of Labor, Mine Safety and Health Administration, Office of Injury and Employment Information, IR 1216.

MSHA [1993e]. Surface stone mine, ID 40–00102, Vulcan Materials Co., Davidson County, TN. Arlington, VA: U.S. Department of Labor, Mine Safety and Health Administration.

MSHA [1994a]. Injury experience in metallic mineral mining, 1993. Denver, CO: U.S. Department of Labor, Mine Safety and Health Administration, Office of Injury and Employment Information, IR 1226.

MSHA [1994b]. Injury experience in nonmetal mineral mining (except stone and coal), 1993. Denver, CO: U.S. Department of Labor, Mine Safety and Health Administration, Office of Injury and Employment Information, IR 1227.

MSHA [1994c]. Injury experience in sand and gravel mining, 1993. Denver, CO: U.S. Department of Labor, Mine Safety and Health Administration, Office of Injury and Employment Information, IR 1229.

MSHA [1994d]. Injury experience in stone mining, 1993. Denver, CO: U.S. Department of Labor, Mine Safety and Health Administration, Office of Injury and Employment Information, IR 1228.

MSHA [1994e]. Metal mill, ID 26–01089, Barrick Goldstrike Mines, Inc., Eureka County, NV. Arlington, VA: U.S. Department of Labor, Mine Safety and Health Administration.

MSHA [1995a]. Injury experience in metallic mineral mining, 1994. Denver, CO: U.S. Department of Labor, Mine Safety and Health Administration, Office of Injury and Employment Information, IR 1233.

MSHA [1995b]. Injury experience in nonmetal mineral mining (except stone and coal), 1994. Denver, CO: U.S. Department of Labor, Mine Safety and Health Administration, Office of Injury and Employment Information, IR 1234.

MSHA [1995c]. Injury experience in sand and gravel mining, 1994. Denver, CO: U.S. Department of Labor, Mine Safety and Health Administration, Office of Injury and Employment Information, IR 1235.

MSHA [1995d]. Injury experience in stone mining, 1994. Denver, CO: U.S. Department of Labor, Mine Safety and Health Administration, Office of Injury and Employment Information, IR 1236.

MSHA [1995e]. Surface metal mine, ID 26–01089, Barrick Goldstrike Mines, Inc., Eureka County, NV. Arlington, VA: U.S. Department of Labor, Mine Safety and Health Administration.

MSHA [1996a]. Injury experience in metallic mineral mining, 1995. Denver, CO: U.S. Department of Labor, Mine Safety and Health Administration, Office of Injury and Employment Information, IR 1243.

MSHA [1996b]. Injury experience in nonmetal mineral mining (except stone and coal), 1995. Denver, CO: U.S. Department of Labor, Mine Safety and Health Administration, Office of Injury and Employment Information, IR 1244.

MSHA [1996c]. Injury experience in sand and gravel mining, 1995. Denver, CO: U.S. Department of Labor, Mine Safety and Health Administration, Office of Injury and Employment Information, IR 1246.

MSHA [1996d]. Injury experience in stone mining, 1995. Denver, CO: U.S. Department of Labor, Mine Safety and Health Administration, Office of Injury and Employment Information, IR 1245.

MSHA [1996e]. Surface sand and gravel mine, ID 42–01828, Christensen Sand and Gravel Co., Cache County, UT. Arlington, VA: U.S. Department of Labor, Mine Safety and Health Administration.

MSHA [1997a]. Injury experience in metallic mineral mining, 1996. Denver, CO: U.S. Department of Labor, Mine Safety and Health Administration, Office of Injury and Employment Information, IR 1254.

MSHA [1997b]. Injury experience in nonmetal mineral mining (except stone and coal), 1996. Denver, CO: U.S. Department of Labor, Mine Safety and Health Administration, Office of Injury and Employment Information, IR 1255.

MSHA [1997c]. Injury experience in sand and gravel mining, 1996. Denver, CO: U.S. Department of Labor, Mine Safety and Health Administration, Office of Injury and Employment Information, IR 1257.

MSHA [1997d]. Injury experience in stone mining, 1996. Denver, CO: U.S. Department of Labor, Mine Safety and Health Administration, Office of Injury and Employment Information, IR 1256.

MSHA [1997e]. Surface metal mine, ID 26–01621, Independence Mining Co., Elko County, NV. Arlington, VA: U.S. Department Of Labor, Mine Safety and Health Administration.

MSHA [1997f]. Underground nonmetal mine, ID 20–00378, G–P Gypsum Corp., Kent County, MI. Arlington, VA: U.S. Department of Labor, Mine Safety and Health Administration.

MSHA [1998a]. Injury experience in metallic mineral mining, 1997. Denver, CO: U.S. Department of Labor, Mine Safety and Health Administration, Office of Injury and Employment Information, IR 1261.

MSHA [1998b]. Injury experience in nonmetal mineral mining (except stone and coal), 1997. Denver, CO: U.S. Department of Labor, Mine Safety and Health Administration, Office of Injury and Employment Information, IR 1262.

MSHA [1998c]. Injury experience in sand and gravel mining, 1997. Denver, CO: U.S. Department of Labor, Mine Safety and Health Administration, Office of Injury and Employment Information, IR 1259.

MSHA [1998d]. Injury experience in stone mining, 1997. Denver, CO: U.S. Department of Labor, Mine Safety and Health Administration, Office of Injury and Employment Information, IR 1260.

MSHA [1999a]. Injury experience in metallic mineral mining, 1998. Denver, CO: U.S. Department of Labor, Mine Safety and Health Administration, Office of Injury and Employment Information, IR 1266.

MSHA [1999b]. Injury experience in nonmetal mineral mining (except stone and coal), 1998. Denver, CO: U.S. Department of Labor, Mine Safety and Health Administration, Office of Injury and Employment Information, IR 1267.

52

MSHA [1999c]. Injury experience in sand and gravel mining, 1998. Denver, CO: U.S. Department of Labor, Mine Safety and Health Administration, Office of Injury and Employment Information, IR 1269.

MSHA [1999d]. Injury experience in stone mining, 1998. Denver, CO: U.S. Department of Labor, Mine Safety and Health Administration, Office of Injury and Employment Information, IR 1268.

MSHA [2000a]. Injury experience in metallic mineral mining, 1999. Denver, CO: U.S. Department of Labor, Mine Safety and Health Administration, Office of Injury and Employment Information, IR 1273.

MSHA [2000b]. Injury experience in nonmetal mineral mining (except stone and coal), 1999. Denver, CO: U.S. Department of Labor, Mine Safety and Health Administration, Office of Injury and Employment Information, IR 1274.

MSHA [2000c]. Injury experience in sand and gravel mining, 1999. Denver, CO: U.S. Department of Labor, Mine Safety and Health Administration, Office of Injury and Employment Information, IR 1276.

MSHA [2000d]. Injury experience in stone mining, 1999. Denver, CO: U.S. Department of Labor, Mine Safety and Health Administration, Office of Injury and Employment Information, IR 1275.

MSHA [2000e]. Surface metal mine, ID 21–01600, Hibbing Taconite Co., St. Louis County, MN. Arlington, VA: U.S. Department of Labor, Mine Safety and Health Administration.

MSHA [2001a]. Injury experience in metallic mineral mining, 2000. Denver, CO: U.S. Department of Labor, Mine Safety and Health Administration, Office of Injury and Employment Information, IR 1280.

MSHA [2001b]. Injury experience in nonmetal mineral mining (except stone and coal), 2000. Denver, CO: U.S. Department of Labor, Mine Safety and Health Administration, Office of Injury and Employment Information, IR 1281.

MSHA [2001c]. Injury experience in sand and gravel mining, 2000. Denver, CO: U.S. Department of Labor, Mine Safety and Health Administration, Office of Injury and Employment Information, IR 1283.

MSHA [2001d]. Injury experience in stone mining, 2000. Denver, CO: U.S. Department of Labor, Mine Safety and Health Administration, Office of Injury and Employment Information, IR 1282.

MSHA [2002a]. Injury experience in metallic mineral mining, 2001. Denver, CO: U.S. Department of Labor, Mine Safety and Health Administration, Office of Injury and Employment Information, IR 1303.

MSHA [2002b]. Injury experience in nonmetal mineral mining (except stone and coal), 2001. Denver, CO: U.S. Department of Labor, Mine Safety and Health Administration, Office of Injury and Employment Information, IR 1304.

MSHA [2002c]. Injury experience in sand and gravel mining, 2001. Denver, CO: U.S. Department of Labor, Mine Safety and Health Administration, Office of Injury and Employment Information, IR 1305.

MSHA [2002d]. Injury experience in stone mining, 2001. Denver, CO: U.S. Department of Labor, Mine Safety and Health Administration, Office of Injury and Employment Information, IR 1306.